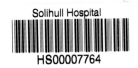

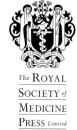

The ROYAL
SOCIETY of
MEDICINE
PRESS Limited

MRSA

in Practice

Ian M Gould

BSc MBChB PhD FRCP(E) FRCPath

Consultant Clinical Microbiologist at
Aberdeen Royal Infirmary, Aberdeen, UK and
Honorary Professor of Public Health,
Epidemiology and Microbiology at the
University of Trnava, Trnava, Slovakia

British Library Cataloguing in Publication Data
A catalogue record for this book is available from the British Library

ISBN 1-85315-687-6
ISSN 1473-6845

Distribution in Europe and Rest of World:
Marston Book Services Ltd
PO Box 269
Abingdon
Oxon OX14 4YN, UK
Tel: +44 (0) 1235 465 500
Fax: +44 (0) 1235 465 555
Email: direct.order@marston.com

Distribution in Australia and New Zealand:
Elsevier Australia
30–52 Smidmore Street
Marrickville NSW 2204
Australia
Tel: + 61 2 9517 8999
Fax: + 61 2 9517 2249
Email: service@elsevier.com.au

Distribution in the USA and Canada:
Royal Society of Medicine Press Ltd
c/o BookMasters, Inc
30 Amberwood Parkway
Ashland, Ohio 44805, USA
Tel: +1 800 247 6553 / +1 800 266 5564
Fax: +1 419 281 6883
E-mail: order@bookmasters.com

Typeset by Phoenix Photosetting, Chatham, Kent
Printed and bound in Spain by Liberdúplex

Preface

I am delighted to have been asked by the Royal Society of Medicine to assemble chapters by such a distinguished group of international experts on MRSA. This book comes at an important crossroad, not only in the development of potential strategies to control MRSA and in the evolution of MRSA clones around the world but also in the development of new antibiotics to combat it.

MRSA is, of course, only one of many different multiresistant microbial pathogens that plague modern-day healthcare systems. All are inevitable consequences of the over-heavy reliance on antibiotics of the past half century, which has selected out MRSA from susceptible staphylococci. Worse still, our attitudes to hygiene have also changed as infectious diseases were thought to be beaten by antibiotics. Certainly, many of our hospitals have seen deteriorating standards of hygiene and cleanliness which have allowed MRSA to spread widely, causing a great deal of professional and public concern and much cost, suffering and death.

I have been fortunate in finding experts to comment on most of these issues and give their visions on an often frightening future. MRSA touches all aspects of modern healthcare and yet there is still a large amount of misunderstanding amongst many doctors about its real significance and how to control it. Some even think it still not worth controlling although it is a huge additional burden to health services around the world. Some think it is just one of many multiresistant organisms to be tackled. Yet MRSA, as this book convincingly shows, is unique in its scale, adaptability and danger to man. It is certainly the largest infection problem to ever trouble modern, developed healthcare services and is now also causing major concerns in selected communities.

After illuminating chapters on the history, pathogenesis and microbiology of MRSA, there are clear chapters on its clinical implications, strategies to control it and how and when to treat it. As with other books in this series, these chapters are written by experts, for their colleagues at the front line who have to deal with the clinical implications of MRSA on a daily basis. At a time when the public and many governments and healthcare administrators are extremely concerned about these issues, I hope that this book is a useful addition to the medical literature, setting MRSA in the context of modern healthcare and improving our knowledge of how to deal with it.

About the editor

Ian M Gould BSc MBChB PhD FRCP(E) FRCPath

Dr Gould is Consultant Clinical Microbiologist at Aberdeen Royal Infirmary and Honorary Professor of Public Health, Epidemiology and Microbiology at the University of Trnava. He trained in clinical microbiology and infectious diseases in the UK, Canada and Africa. Dr Gould is Editor or Board member of several international journals and Chairman, Secretary or council member of various national/international working parties, learned societies and advisory boards on antibiotic policies and resistance. He is advisor on antibiotic resistance and prescribing to the UK Department of Health, Alliance for the Prudent Use of Antibiotics, The International Organisation for Epizoonosis, European Commission, The European Centre for Disease Control and government agencies abroad. He was co-ordinator of the European projects ESAR and ARPAC. Dr Gould has 200 published scientific papers on antibiotic policies and resistance in peer-reviewed journals, standard texts and specialist books. He is founder of the International Working Group on MRSA (<www.ischemo.org>).

Contents

Introduction 1
Ian M Gould

1 MRSA: a historical perspective 3
Ian Phillips

Methicillin 4
MRSA – resistant or not? 4
MRSA – epidemic or not? 6
MRSA – singular and plural 7
MRSA – multiresistant, virulent and epidemic 7
Control 9
Treatment 9
Lessons from the past 10
Conclusions 11

2 Pathogenesis and immunology of MSSA and MRSA carriage and infection 13
Alex van Belkum

Infectious syndromes caused by S. aureus 13
Virulence factors of S. aureus 14
Innate immune evasion 15
Humoral immunity 16
Cellular immunity 16
Mucosal colonisation and local inflammatory responses 16
Interference therapy, passive immunotherapy and vaccines 17
Are MRSA more virulent or invoking different immune responses than MSSA? 17
Conclusions 18

3 The evolution of MRSA 21
Ben R D Short, Mark C Enright

Early MRSA 21
Investigating the evolution of MRSA 21
Evolutionary mechanisms 23
Evolutionary history of MRSA 23
Concluding remarks 27

4 Epidemiology of MRSA 29
Jaana Vuopio-Varkila

Variation in MRSA rates 29

Geographic variation 30
MRSA situation in specific countries 30
MRSA carriage 31
Surveillance 32
MRSA and outbreaks 33

5 MRSA at home and on the farm 37
Andreas Voss, Margreet C Vos

Defining non-healthcare acquired MRSA 37
Epidemiology 39
Prevention of CA-MRSA and CO-MRSA 41
MRSA in animals 42

6 MRSA – advances in laboratory detection, identification and antibiotic susceptibility testing 49
Donald Morrison

Rapid MRSA laboratory reporting 49
Molecular basis of methicillin resistance 50
Laboratory detection and confirmation of MRSA 51
Conclusions 57

7 Antibiotic resistance in MRSA 59
Giles Edwards

Patterns of resistance 59
β-Lactams 60
Glycopeptides 61
Other antibiotics 62
Future trends 65

8 Clinical features of community-acquired MRSA 67
Tristan Ferry, Jerome Etienne

CA-MRSA skin and soft tissue infections 68
CA-MRSA pulmonary infections 68
CA-MRSA bone and joint infections 69
Other CA-MRSA organ infections 69
CA-MRSA bacteraemia and disseminated infections 69
CA-MRSA septic shock and purpura fulminans 69

Diagnosis of CA-MRSA infections   70
General recommendations for patients with
   CA-MRSA infections   70

9   **Clinical presentation of MRSA
    infections**   71
    Hisham Ziglam, Dilip Nathwani

Colonisation and infection   71
Infections associated with MRSA   73
Skin and soft-tissue infection   73
MRSA bacteraemia   73
MRSA endocarditis   74
MRSA and bone infection   75
Hospital/ventilator acquired pneumonia   75
MRSA and postoperative infections   76
Conclusions   76

10   **Treatment of MRSA infection**   79
     Ian M Gould, Abhijit M Bal

Antibiotics for treatment of MRSA infection   80
Practical considerations in the treatment of
   MRSA   83
Screening for MRSA carriage and
   decontamination   84

11   **Decolonisation of MRSA patients**   87
     R Andrew Seaton

The consequences of MRSA colonisation   87
Agents used to decolonise patients with
   MRSA   88
Is it possible to eradicate MRSA
   colonisation?   89
Is it possible to prevent MRSA infection through
   decolonisation strategies?   89
How should MRSA-colonised patients be
   managed?   90

12   **Alternative treatments for MRSA**   93
     Thomas V Riley

Medicinal plants   94
Essential oils   94
Honey   96
Bacteriophages as antimicrobial agents   96
Bacterial interference   97
Conclusions   98

13   **Mopping up MRSA**   101
     Stephanie J Dancer

Background   101
History of staphylococcal epidemiology   102
Staphylococcal transmission cycle   102
Staphylococcal carriage   103
Airborne transmission   103

Contamination in hospitals   104
Survival of staphylococci   104
Human transmission   104
Dynamic relationship between people and the
   environment regarding staphylococcal
   transmission   105
Effect of cleaning   106
Importance of hand-touch sites   107
Conclusions   107

14   **MRSA control in the community**   109
     Hans Jørn Kolmos

Epidemiology   109
Aim and strategy   111
Detection of MRSA   111
Nursing homes and other long-term care
   facilities   112
Clients receiving home care   113
Schools, kindergartens and day-care
   centres   114
Clinics (medical, dental, physiotherapy,
   pedicure, etc.)   114
Ambulances, taxis and public transport   114
Treatment of MRSA carriers and follow-up   115

15   **The SISS MRSA guidance: risk
     assessment and targeted
     screening**   117
     Dugald Baird

A Scottish perspective   117
Background – a steadily increasing pool of
   colonised patients   118
The SISS guidance   121
Principles of the approach   121
Appendix 1   126
Appendix 2   126

16   **Surveillance of MRSA**   131
     Georgia J Duckworth

Background and definition   132
What does surveillance do?   133
Sources of data   133
Objectives, definitions and dataset   134
Quality of the data   135
Numerators, denominators and analysis of
   the data   135
Recording and monitoring infections   135
Feeding back the data and action   136
Resourcing the surveillance   137
Conclusions   137

Index   141

Contributors

Dugald Baird
Consultant Microbiologist (retired), East
Kilbride, Glasgow, G74 4LA, UK
E-mail: dugalbaird@hotmail.com

Abhijit M Bal
Specialist Registrar, Department of Medical
Microbiology, Aberdeen Royal Infirmary,
Foresterhill, Aberdeen AB25 2ZN, UK
E-mail: a.bal@abdn.ac.uk

Stephanie J Dancer
Consultant Microbiologist, Department of
Microbiology, Southern General Hospital, 1345
Govan Road, Glasgow G51 4TF, UK
E-mail: stephanie.dancer@sgh.scot.nhs.uk

Georgia J Duckworth
Director, Department of Healthcare Associated
Infection & Antimicrobial Resistance, Centre for
Infections, Health Protection Agency – CDSC,
61 Colindale Avenue, London NW9 5EQ, UK
E-mail: georgia.duckworth@hpa.org.uk

Giles Edwards
Consultant Microbiologist, Glasgow Health
Board and Scottish MRSA Reference Laboratory,
Stobhill Hospital, Glasgow G21 3UW, UK
E-mail: Giles.Edwards@northglasgow.scot.nhs.uk

Mark C Enright
Reader in Molecular Epidemiology, Department
of Infectious Disease Epidemiology, Faculty of
Medicine, Imperial College London, Old Medical
School Building, St Mary's Hospital, Norfolk
Place, London W2 1PG, UK
E-mail: m.c.enright@imperial.ac.uk

Jerome Etienne
Laboratoire de Bactériologie, INSERM E0230,
IFR62, Faculté de Médecine Laennec, Rue
Guillaume Paradin, F-69372 Lyon cedex 08,
France
E-mail jetienne@univ-lyon1.fr

Tristan Ferry
Laboratoire de Bactériologie, INSERM E0230,
IFR62, Faculté de Médecine Laennec, Rue
Guillaume Paradin, F-69372 Lyon cedex 08,
France
E-mail: tristan.ferry@univ-lyon1.fr

Ian M Gould
Consultant Microbiologist, Aberdeen Royal
Infirmary, Foresterhill, Aberdeen AB25 2ZN, UK
E-mail: i.m.gould@abdn.ac.uk

Hans Jørn Kolmos
Professor of Microbiology, University of
Southern Denmark, Consultant Microbiologist,
Department of Clinical Microbiology, Odense
University Hospital, Winsløwparken 21, 2nd
Floor, DK-5000 Odense C, Denmark
E-mail: hans.joern.kolmos@ouh.fyns-amt.dk

Donald Morrison
Principal Clinical Scientist, Scottish MRSA
Reference Laboratory, Microbiology Department,
Stobhill Hospital, Glasgow G21 3UW, UK
E-mail: donald.morrison@northglasgow.scot.nhs.uk

Dilip Nathwani
Consultant Physician, Infection Unit, East
Block, Ninewells Hospital, Dundee DD1 9SY, UK
E-mail: dilip.nathwani@tuht.scot.nhs.uk

Ian Phillips
Emeritus Professor of Microbiology, Guy's and St
Thomas's Hospitals Medical School, London, UK

Thomas V Riley
Professor of Microbiology and Immunology, The
University of Western Australia and Division of
Microbiology and Infectious Diseases, PathWest
Laboratory Medicine, Queen Elizabeth II Medical
Centre, Nedlands 6009, Western Australia,
Australia
E-mail: triley@cyllene.uwa.edu.au

R Andrew Seaton
Consultant Physician (Infectious Diseases and
General Medicine), Brownlee Centre, Gartnavel
General Hospital, 1053 Great Western Road,
Glasgow G12 0YN, UK
E-mail:
andrew.seaton@northglasgow.scot.nhs.uk

Ben R D Short
Research Assistant, Department of Infectious
Disease Epidemiology, Faculty of Medicine,
Imperial College London, Old Medical School
Building, St Mary's Hospital, Norfolk Place,
London W2 1PG, UK

Alex van Belkum
Department of Medical Microbiology and
Infectious Diseases, Erasmus Medical Centre, Dr
Molewaterplein 40, NL-3015 GD Rotterdam, The
Netherlands
E-mail: a.vanbelkum@erasmusmc.nl

Margreet C Vos
Medical Microbiologist and Head Infection
Control, Department of Medical Microbiology
and Infectious Diseases, Erasmus Medical
Centre, Dr Moleewaterplein 40, 3015 GD
Rotterdam, The Netherlands
E-mail: m.vos@erasmusmc.nl

Andreas Voss
Professor of Infection Control, Radboud
University Nijmegen Medical Centre, Nijmegen
and Clinical Microbiologist and Head Infection
Control, Canisius-Wilhelmina Hospital,
Department of Medical Microbiology (C-70),
PO Box, 6500 GS Nijmegen, The Netherlands
E-mail: vossandreas@gmail.com

Jaana Vuopio-Varkila
Chief Physician, Hospital Bacteria Laboratory,
National Public Health Institute,
Mannerheimintie 166, 00300 Helsinki, Finland
E:mail: jaana.vuopio@ktl.fi

Hisham Ziglam
Senior Registrar in Infectious Diseases
Infection Unit, East Block, Ninewells Hospital,
Dundee DD1 9SY, UK
E:mail: hisham.ziglam@taht.scot.nhs.uk

Introduction

Ian M Gould

Methicillin-resistant *Staphylococcus aureus* (MRSA) is the most important of the superbugs that have arisen since the advent of antibiotics. It poses a huge threat to health services world-wide most of which have shown little resolve to deal with it effectively. While natural evolution suggests some hope for regression in virulence, there is no evidence as yet of that actually happening. Indeed, new, even more virulent clones are arising in the community, often highly transmissible, capable of causing life-threatening disease in healthy young people and even invading hospitals and supplanting the older strains of MRSA derived originally from the hospital itself.

Methicillin, the first of the semi-synthetic penicillins, was developed by Beecham laboratories in the late 1950s to combat the then scourge of β-lactamase producing, tetracycline and streptomycin resistant clones that were causing havoc in many hospitals around the world. While resistance to it first evolved in 1961, MRSA did not really become important clinically, on a world-wide basis, until the mid to late 1980s; the problem has got progressively worse since then as new more transmissible and more virulent clones have evolved sequentially.

After much debate about possible clinical significance, it is increasingly accepted by many (but not all) doctors that MRSA is a major clinical issue. Depending upon the strain, mortality can be double that of a corresponding infection with an antibiotic-susceptible strain, length of stay for survivors at least double, and

morbidity extensive. Recent estimates suggest a huge excess cost to the tax payer as MRSA is an additional burden to health services and not just a replacement of more antibiotic susceptible infections.

Unfortunately, there are not many robust statistics on the real costs of MRSA to healthcare systems and society but data from the UK, which has one of the highest rates in Europe and from the US, which has one of the highest rates in the world, suggest the costs are huge. Bloodstream infections (bacteraemia) with MRSA have been notifiable for several years now in the UK and there are currently approximately 10,000 episodes per year. The mortality rate of MRSA bacteraemia is 40–50% and the attributable mortality probably about 20%; so, this represents a huge number of deaths. Many serious infections with MRSA are not counted in these figures because blood cultures are not taken or, for one reason or another, were not positive. Many of these infections will also be fatal, many others will lead to chronic morbidity, especially from incurable prosthetic infections, particularly orthopaedic implants.

The costs, just of extended stay in hospital, are now measured in billions of pounds or dollars per year in the UK and US, respectively. In the US, the extra healthcare insurance costs have been estimated at $30 billion per year and in the UK a decline in GDP of over £10 billion per year has been estimated. Paradoxically, there is still a wide-spread ambivalence about the significance of MRSA, with much doubt about the advisability of spending scarce resources on its control. However, while these huge sums are alarming, they could get much worse if nothing is done.

At the moment there is great debate in public health circles about the advisability of spending on major control efforts, although all the evidence is consistent that they would work, controlling MRSA in the UK within 5 years, at a cost of up to several hundred million pounds. The money will need to be spent mainly on case identification and strict isolation of MRSA carriers while in hospital, which will necessitate much better facilities in many hospitals than currently exist. However, much of the money spent will be a one-off, money well spent and reaping benefits for many years to come. The basic principles will also stand us in good stead for the control of many other infections, including the frightening evolutionary consequences of further variants of MRSA such as vancomycin-resistant strains and community-acquired MRSA (CA-MRSA).

In many ways, CA-MRSA, which is already with us in many communities around the world, is even more frightening. While not as multiply antibiotic resistant as hospital-acquired MRSA, it tends to be laden with many more toxins and super antigens, allowing the development of particularly aggressive soft-tissue and lung infections, such as necrotising fasciitis and haemorrhagic pneumonia. It can spread very rapidly around family and close community groups and is showing worrying tendencies to evolve further into more antibiotic resistant strains and spread within hospitals. It is even less clear how to stop its spread in the community than it is how we are to control hospital MRSA.

What does the future hold? Probably a never ending battle with the wily staphylococcus. Probably a never ending battle with the politicians and healthcare administrators to spend the necessary resources on the problem. At the moment, short-termism seems to rule in cash-strapped hospitals and arguments that money spent today will save much more next year seem to have limited impact. Public

anxiety and loss of confidence in our hospitals has had some effect but these advances need to be consolidated and multiplied many fold if we are to win the current battle with MRSA, never mind the war.

Future hospitals will need to be at least 50% single-room occupancy. Scandinavia, which has kept relatively clear of MRSA up till now by a 'seek and destroy' policy, is now building 100% single-room occupancy. We need to rediscover the cleanliness regimens that Florence Nightingale introduced and which we lost when we were lulled into a false sense of security by the advent of the antibiotic era. We must stimulate much more research into new antibiotics and into learning the weaknesses and strength of the staphylococcus so that we can out manoeuvre it, perhaps with vaccines, perhaps with immune modulators or phage therapy, perhaps by so-far undreamt of means. The effort will be worth it. The staphylococcus is, so far, unique amongst micro-organisms in its combination of epidemiology, pathogenicity, transmissibility and virulence. Lets hope it stays that way!

Two further thoughts: *Staphylococcus pneumoniae* was probably a major cause of death in young people during the 1918 flu pandemic. If there is another flu pandemic and we have done nothing to control the spread of toxin-loaded CA-MRSA, particularly PVL positive strains which are associated with haemorrhagic pneumonia, then we are likely to see the same problems again with high mortality.

Second, Alexander Ogston, Professor of Surgery at Aberdeen in the late 1800s and the discoverer of the staphylococcus and its importance in surgical sepsis was able to remove the sign above his ward 'Prepare to meet thy maker' when he introduced Listerian concepts of antisepsis. Up until that time, mortality from sepsis after major surgery was probably at least 50%. To the public it must often now seem that the days of the hospital as a disease maker have returned. The medical profession owes it to them to make sure this situation is rapidly reversed.

1. MRSA: a historical perspective

Ian Phillips

Methicillin
MRSA – resistant or not?
MRSA – epidemic or not?
MRSA – singular and plural
MRSA – multiresistant, virulent and
  epidemic
Control
Treatment
Lessons from the past
Conclusions

It is always difficult to know when history ends and current affairs begin. I have taken the relevant period to be the late 1950s to the early 1990s, three and a half decades in which I was at first a clinical medical student in London (in the days when it was customary to separate pre-clinical and clinical studies) and latterly a consultant medical microbiologist, up to the time when administrative duties finally removed me from direct involvement in clinical microbiology. During this time, methicillin-resistant *Staphylococcus aureus* (MRSA) evolved from being a laboratory curiosity to become a major public health threat.

The first description of the then new β-lactam antibiotic methicillin appeared in 1959 and this was soon followed by reports of methicillin resistance in clinical isolates of *S. aureus*. The mechanism of this acquired resistance was soon shown not to involve staphylococcal β-lactamases, to which the drug was stable, and because of this and the rarity of MRSA, it was initially widely believed that they had little clinical significance.

Much of the early action in relation to MRSA centred on London. One can point to a number of circumstances that may explain this. Methicillin was the product of the Beecham Research Laboratories, an institution that had much more of the flavour of a university department rather than a commercial establishment. These laboratories were at Brockham Park, only a few miles south of London. The London hospitals were in their heyday, with a dozen undergraduate teaching hospitals, as many postgraduate teaching hospitals, and a plethora of other independent or associated hospitals. It was relatively easy to congregate a dozen professors of microbiology from the area, many of whom had dealt with *Streptococcus pyogenes* before and during the Second World War, and had gone on to deal with the problem of increasing antibiotic resistance of *S. aureus* in their associated hospital wards. Finally, the Public Health Laboratory Service's Staphylococcal and Streptococcal Reference Laboratory, which took the lead in developing phage typing of *S. aureus*, was at Colindale in the northern suburbs of London. At a time when the means of communication were decidedly less well developed than they are today, this concentration of patients, doctors and scientists, with a talented team of drug developers on their doorstep, was well able to tackle MRSA.

The earliest methicillin-resistant isolates were first reported as 'Celbenin'-resistant – relating to the proprietary name of the first penicillinase-resistant penicillin developed and marketed by Beecham – and only subsequently as methicillin-resistant *S. aureus*, or MRSA. A confusion of acronyms subsequently arose as new anti-staphylococcal penicillins were introduced, such as oxacillin (the first of a series of isoxazolyl penicillins), which led to the use of the acronym ORSA in some parts of the world. However, a paradox soon arose when the clinical use of methicillin was largely abandoned as improved derivatives became available, but MRSA persisted as the usual name, somewhat to the confusion of later generations of students and clinicians. When it became clear that MRSA were resistant to all clinically available penicillins, cephalosporins and later penems they might have been called β-lactam-resistant *S. aureus* – βLRSA perhaps – but no such suggestion was made to my knowledge, although the paradox was noted.[1]

> 'Initial studies five years ago led some of us to predict that the emergence of methicillin-resistant staphylococci would not become a problem. This ... now appears to have been correct.'
>
> Kirby (1964)[2]

Despite early prognostications, MRSA has indeed posed problems to microbiologists, epidemiologists and clinicians, and has often behaved in a paradoxical way. As will be seen from the contributions to this volume, not all the problems have been solved.

Methicillin

Methicillin was one of the early group of antibiotics whose production was made possible by the discovery, and then the biosynthesis, of 6-aminopenicillanic acid, the backbone of the penicillins.[3,4] It was suitable for the treatment of infections caused by penicillin-resistant staphylococci because it was resistant to staphylococcal β-lactamase, but not to acid (and could thus not be administered orally).[4,5] Eventually, as recorded by George Rolinson in his Garrod Lecture, a number of compounds resistant to staphylococcal β-lactamase, with or without acid stability, and with greater potency than methicillin, became available.[4]

Methicillin was rapidly shown to be effective for the treatment of infections in experimental animals[6] and treatment and prevention of staphylococcal infections in humans.[7–9] Other derivatives equally rapidly followed.[2,9] The speed of progress from new chemical entity to availability to clinicians will seem remarkable to those who now have to wait for years for the same progression! Expectations of methicillin

and its successors were justifiably high, since hospital staphylococci had, by the late 1950s, cumulated resistance to penicillin, streptomycin, chloramphenicol, tetracyclines, erythromycin, novobiocin and finally kanamycin, soon after they were, in turn, introduced. Since fusidic acid, rifampicin and co-trimoxazole had not yet appeared, vancomycin was the only antibiotic available, and was indeed used despite its disadvantages. We were saved by the bell!

> 'A penicillin resistant to staphylococcal penicillinase (may) finally silence the adaptable staphylococcus'.
>
> Barber (1961)[10]

One interesting early use of methicillin in prevention was reported by Steven Elek of St George's Hospital (then at Hyde Park Corner in the building now occupied by a luxury hotel) in 1960.[11] Based on the finding that nasal carriage and dispersal from the noses of patients and staff were important in the dissemination of infection, he introduced the spraying of methicillin in wards. This was strikingly effective in controlling staphylococcal infection: nasal carriage was virtually abolished as was environmental contamination, and all staphylococcal infections occurred in patients in unsprayed wards.[10] As may be imagined, some were dismayed by such usage but, despite predictions, no methicillin-resistant *S. aureus* emerged (although methicillin-resistant 'micrococci' did, but caused no trouble), and a few others followed suit with similar results.[12,13] When it became clear that clinically relevant MRSA were more than a theoretical possibility, the practice stopped.

MRSA – resistant or not?

The first report of MRSA came from Dr Tom Parker and his staff, notably Patricia Jevons, in the Public Health Reference Laboratory at Colindale. They were probably the first to see small staphylococcal colonies growing in very small numbers within a normal or only slightly reduced zone of inhibition of growth around methicillin-containing discs on lawns of staphylococcal growth. These naturally resistant strains were quite different from those developed in the laboratory by serial passage on increasing concentrations of the drug.[10,14] Such clinical strains accounted for a very small number of over 5000 isolates of *S. aureus*, largely from south-east England, sent to them in late 1960 for phage typing because they were resistant to other antibiotics.[15] By the techniques used at the time, methicillin minimum inhibitory concentrations (MICs) were often only marginally higher than those for susceptible strains – susceptible strains were inhibited by 1.25–2.5 mg/l while resistant strains required 3.12–25 mg/l – and it is possible that not all resistant strains were detected.[15,16] Mary Barber reported that she had found a single isolate of MRSA among the first 500 staphylococcal isolates that she screened at the Hammersmith Hospital.[10]

The determination of MICs of methicillin, for a range of inocula of MRSA, soon showed that these cultures contained large numbers of bacterial cells slightly more methicillin resistant than normal, and diminishing numbers resistant to successively higher concentrations of the drug, thus providing a definition of heteroresistance.[16,17] Since they did not destroy methicillin, Barber referred to them as 'tolerant',[10] a term now used quite differently. Similar strains were subsequently isolated in many laboratories in Europe and beyond.[18,19] By 1964, the Colindale laboratory had screened almost 45,000 staphylococcal isolates submitted for phage typing and detected MRSA from 35 mostly UK laboratories, suggesting that they were usually endemic rather than epidemic.[19] It seems possible that heteroresistance was already diminishing since they described some strains as 'growing up to the disc'.[19]

Since MRSA clearly existed before methicillin was widely used and, furthermore, often failed to appear in many hospitals in which it was intensively used, the exact antibiotic providing

selecting pressure was, and often is, not clear. Indeed, MRSA were reported where no methicillin had been used – in Delhi, where Pal and his colleagues found that 12% of staphylococcal infections in adults and neonates in the All India Institute of Medical Sciences Hospital were caused by MRSA and carriage was not uncommon,[20] and in Gdansk where a still surprising 50% of mothers and babies in one hospital were carriers.[21]

'We identified our first strain, retrospectively because of difficulties in detecting methicillin resistance, from a minor skin lesion of a patient in an obstetrics ward in April 1962'.

Cookson and Phillips (1990)[22]

It remained doubtful that these highly heteroresistant strains might be clinically significant, or might be a hazard to the efficacy of methicillin. One of my first laboratory studies as a trainee microbiologist was to re-test stored isolates and discover a handful of MRSA, none of which had been recognised at the time of their isolation as being clinically or microbiologically resistant.[22] The infections, at least in some cases, were not trivial, and I remember in particular a patient with acute osteomyelitis for whom surgical intervention had presumably been a major determinant of a successful outcome, possibly aided by methicillin. In total, MRSA was isolated, and identified retrospectively, from the lesions of 15 more patients in nine different wards in St Thomas's Hospital in 1962–1963, with little evidence of cross-infection.[22] However, one hospital stood out against the rule, the paediatric hospital Queen Mary's, Carshalton, a few miles south of London. Methicillin use, including limited ward spraying, had started in the hospital in 1959, but MRSA were not seen until 1961 when two patients were found to be nasal carriers, following which a clear outbreak of infection affected 37 children. Subsequently, there were more infections and a child operated on for spina bifida developed a wound infection and then septicaemia and died. Here, there was no doubt as to the clinical significance of MRSA and of its ability to colonise and cross-infect susceptible children.[13]

Clearly, it was necessary that techniques be developed for the efficient detection of MRSA in diagnostic laboratories. Tests on large inocula in liquid media (broth macrodilution in those days), which did detect them, were not suitable for routine use. Mary Barber reported that protection from lysis by 'osmotic support', achievable, for example, by increasing the concentration of sodium chloride in the broth or in the agar plate, very much reduced the degree of heteroresistance.[18] A commercially available medium, mannitol-salt agar (Chapman's medium) had a similar effect, as well as demonstrating that the organism was indeed *S. aureus* and not a coagulase-negative staphylococcus, of little clinical significance at that time. Annear in Australia demonstrated that growth at a lower temperature than the 37°C normally used, also allowed the more sensitive moiety to grow in higher concentrations of methicillin, recommending an incubation temperature of 30–35°C.[23] The scene was set for the ready detection of these strains, later aided by the development of genetic probes and other genetic methods discussed elsewhere in this book.

MRSA – epidemic or not?

Initially, despite some rather striking exceptions, MRSA fulfilled expectations and remained rare; indeed, the use of methicillin seemed to have only a minor epidemiological effect. Mary Barber argued both ways and recommended caution!

'It was unwise to assume that the staphylococcus had met its match'.

Barber (1961)[19]

At the Colindale reference laboratory, MRSA accounted for only 0.06–0.29% of isolates sent for phage typing between 1960 and 1962, excluding isolates from the paediatric hospital

that uniquely suffered cross-infection.[19] In St Thomas's Hospital, after the initial flurry of isolates, MRSA completely disappeared for 2 years in the face of extensive use of methicillin and, subsequently, cloxacillin. After this period, MRSA returned, but did not account for more than 2% per annum of isolates in the hospital; between 1975 and 1978, they accounted for less than 0.4% of isolates.[22] Others had similar experiences. Chabbert reported from the Institut Pasteur reference laboratory in Paris that, although no strains were isolated before 1960, 10 isolates of MRSA were identified from nine Paris hospitals in late 1961 and early 1962. These strains had been submitted because patients were failing to respond to antibiotics.[24] Oddly, in the US and Canada, according to Fleming's statement in discussion following a paper by Mary Barber at a conference in London in 1964, no MRSA were detected in the earliest years.[18] Again she had warned that things might change, invoking what Tom Parker called Barber's Law, which drew attention to the interaction of antibiotic use and cross-infection in hospitals in the genesis of the multiply antibiotic-resistant hospital staphylococcus. Sadly, Mary Barber was killed in a car crash in 1965, and the 'slim figure with short, straight unadorned hair ... well known as a forceful speaker and formidable opponent in debate', as described by Paul Garrod in her obituary notice in the *British Medical Journal*, was greatly missed. She had had a central role in studies of the evolution of the multiresistant 'Hospital Staphylococcus' and of the early MRSA.

'If there is widespread use (of penicillinase-resistant penicillins) in wards where cross-infection is occurring, drug resistance might once more become a problem'.

Barber (1962)[25]

Over time, as she half predicted, increases in prevalence started to appear in different parts of the world. Richard Wenzel and his colleagues documented their appearance in Europe, Australia, Africa, the Middle East, and Asia as well as in the US.[26] In Zurich, they accounted for 9.7%, 17.3% and 16.1% of staphylococcal clinical isolates in 1965, 1966 and 1967, respectively.[27] In Denmark, they became unexpectedly prevalent. According to Kirsten Rosendahl of the State Serum Institute, they accounted for 10% of staphylococcal bacteraemia isolates by 1966 and a staggering 46% by 1970.[28] When this very high prevalence was reversed, the diminished use of streptomycin and tetracycline was held responsible, at least in part, but why others had not experienced the problem in such an extreme form at that stage remains a mystery. MRSA remained rare in the US until 1976; however, in the subsequent 5 years, 18 outbreaks were reported. Patients in critical care were especially vulnerable, associated with their long hospital stay and previous antibiotic use.[29]

MRSA – singular and plural

It was a striking finding that all the earliest MRSA belonged to a limited number of phage types of what was known as Group III[15] and had the same antibiotic-resistance pattern – resistant to penicillin, streptomycin and tetracycline (PST). Interestingly, the first penicillin-resistant staphylococci were also lysed by a small number of Group III phages.[30] The three original methicillin-resistant isolates isolated at Colindale all came from one hospital and were of phage type 7/47/53/54/75/77.[15] The St Thomas's isolates of 1962–1963 were invariably of phage type 53/75/77 and also had the PST-resistance pattern.[22] In Paris, they were shown all to belong initially to the same serotype.[24] It was notable that these early strains differed in both phage type and, in a lesser degree, in antibiotic resistance from the 'Hospital Staphylococcus' of the time.[31]

'It has repeatedly been observed that when staphylococci resistant to a particular antibiotic first become prevalent, they have a restricted range of phage typing'.

Parker and Jevons (1964)[19]

A change came quickly. It was very soon clear on the basis of phage typing that other staphylococci, seemingly not closely related to the first clone, were also acquiring methicillin resistance as well as a greater spectrum of multiple antibiotic resistance. For example, in 1964, Parker and Jevons reported that many isolates now did indeed have the characteristics of the descendants of the methicillin-sensitive 80/81 strain that caused the hospital pandemic of the 1950s and 1960s.[19] Furthermore, Chabbert reported French strains additionally resistant to erythromycin, chloramphenicol, and novobiocin in 1962 although they still belonged to phage Group III.[24] We were aware that genetic information was changing hands among *S. aureus* but did not, and could not at the time, understand the means.

In 1980, the mechanism of methicillin resistance was shown to be related to the presence of a low-affinity penicillin-binding protein (PBP),[32] soon shown to be a new protein named either PBP 2a or PBP2'.[33] The *mec* gene responsible, not native to *S. aureus*, was later shown to be carried on the chromosome, but its origin remained obscure.[22] Before long, other genes were shown to be involved,[34] and links with genes responsible for efflux of metal ions and antiseptics were also found.[22] Some Australian strains were resistant to 20 different antibiotics and antiseptics.[35]

The full understanding of the complex evolutionary events taking place was impossible on the basis of the traditional methods of phage- and sero-typing, and had to wait almost 40 years until the appropriate molecular technology had been developed. This is discussed elsewhere in this book.

MRSA – multiresistant, virulent and epidemic

In 1968, Phyllis Rountree (another renowned student of the staphylococci) and her colleagues reported from Sydney a growing problem with MRSA infection from 1965 – the

MRSA being often also resistant to erythromycin and chloramphenicol.[36] By 1979, six of 31 metropolitan hospitals in Victoria found that 20–40% of clinical isolates of *S. aureus* were MRSA.[37] Resistance to gentamicin, fusidic acid and rifampicin was also reported, and many of the isolates were untypable by the normal phage set. There were also reports from Victoria of a resurgence of infections in the newborn in hospitals.[38] Epidemic MRSA, arguably more virulent than the early strains, and now often also resistant to many more antibiotics, had arrived and subsequently appeared in countries around the world.[39]

In the UK, epidemic strains resembled the Australian strains and were soon labelled 'epidemic MRSA' (EMRSA). Some hospitals in the south-east of England had major outbreaks. At the London Hospital, David Williams and his colleagues reported a hard-fought battle against repeated outbreaks involving some 500 patients over a 4-year period.[40] The Royal Free Hospital was also badly affected as were hospitals in Dublin, although the strains there were different.[41] In St Thomas's Hospital, EMRSA suddenly appeared when the MRSA prevalence jumped from 0.2% in 1983 to 11% in 1984, clearly demonstrating their epidemic potential, as well as their difference from what were called 'other' MRSA (OMRSA).[42] Richard Marples and his colleagues at Colindale recognised them as different because of the involvement of large numbers of hospitals, initially mostly in the London area.[43] Some of those who had not yet been caught up in the pandemic, notably Richard Lacey, doubted that these strains differed in any important way from other staphylococci,[44] and it proved difficult to persuade them that special measures might be needed to contain them. Unfortunately, there is still no means of direct detection of the bacterial property that John McGowan and I have called epidemigenicity, and for any new strain one must await events – that is, the detection of epidemics followed by the characterisation of the strains by phenotypic or genotypic means.

> 'If these organisms are remarkable then it is for their failure to spread universally during the 25 years that they have been recognized'.
>
> Lacey (1987)[44]

Other epidemic strains arrived, notably what were called in the UK EMRSA-15 and EMRSA-16,[43] and strains peculiar to Japan and the US;[41] it is only recently that the unravelling of relationships on a global scale has been attempted (see chapter by Ben R D Short and Mark C Enright).

By 1991, the growth of the epidemic over three decades was causing major problems in many parts of the world, including Europe, Australia, Africa, the Middle East, Asia and the US.[26] In the US in the late 1980s, 16–22% of staphylococcal isolates from patients in large hospitals were MRSA, while even smaller hospitals had an incidence of 5–8%.[26] In Europe, the new epidemiological network EARSS, devoted to antibiotic-resistant pathogens, reported that although the prevalence of MRSA still differed widely in different parts of Europe, in some it had reached new heights. During the period 1998–2000, although in Denmark (notably, in view of the earlier high incidence), Finland, Iceland, The Netherlands and Sweden fewer than 2% of isolates from patients with bloodstream infections were MRSA, between 30–40% of bacteraemia isolates in Bulgaria, Spain, Greece, Ireland, Italy, Malta, Portugal and the UK were MRSA.[45] It was noted that patients in ICUs were particularly likely to acquire MRSA infections.

> 'There has been a global epidemic of MRSA in the last three decades'.
>
> Wenzel *et al.* (1991)[26]

> MRSA poses 'therapeutic problems for clinicians, management difficulties for nurses, confusion for infection control practitioners and resource-allocation uncertainties for hospital administrators'.
>
> Mulligan et al. (1993)[46]

> 'How long can intensive levels of surveillance and action be maintained?'
>
> Duckworth and Williams (1988)[40]

Control

In the early years, MRSA rarely caused serious cross-infection in hospitals, but when they did, in most cases they were controlled by the methods that were in common use for multiresistant hospital staphylococci. The results of extensive surveillance[39] showed that the clinical success of the epidemic strains lay in large part in their ability to colonise the hands of members of staff, albeit transiently, rather than to colonise their noses more permanently.[47] Members of staff with skin lesions such as patches of eczema or bitten finger nail beds, did become longer-term carriers, however.[48] In order to cut off this source, it was found to be necessary to isolate and treat patients, sometimes in cohorts,[43] with full precautions against cross-infection and to improve facilities and methods for hand-washing, including the use of alcoholic hand washes.[22,40] In addition, staff carriers were excluded from duty and treated with antiseptics; however, it was not until mupirocin became available for the topical treatment of carrier sites that high rates of success were achieved.[22] A great deal of advice on control was disseminated, none of it fundamentally different from what Mary Barber had preached in the early 1960s, when, incidentally, she also invented antibiotic policies. The frustration of those doing their best to control outbreaks of MRSA infection with inadequate resources, often in the full glare of press, public and political interest seldom emerges from the published accounts, but there were a few cries of pain!

In the UK, a Working Party of the Hospital Infection Society and the British Society for Antimicrobial Chemotherapy issued influential guidelines in 1986 and revised them in 1990.[49,50]

In the 1990s, MRSA spread to nursing homes and residential homes for the elderly, and once again guidelines for the control of this phenomenon were issued.[51] Finally, mention must be made of community isolates of MRSA producing the Panton-Valentine leucocidin, which has been responsible for severe community infections.[52] In earlier days, the toxin was held to be produced by many hospital staphylococci, but little was made of this observation.

Treatment

Before the advent of MRSA, each antibiotic had been lost for the treatment of the 'Hospital Staphylococcus' as resistance accumulated. By the late 1950s, strains resistant to all available antibiotics – that is penicillin, streptomycin, tetracycline, chloramphenicol, erythromycin and novobiocin, but not to vancomycin – were common in hospitals. I well remember the so-called 'Staph' book at St Thomas' Hospital in the early 1960s with no shortage of entries of 'PSTCENv-resistant' in red. Vancomycin thus became the antibiotic of last resort for infections with these strains not long after its introduction in 1956.[39] Initially it was an impure product – referred to as 'Mississippi Mud' – with a high incidence of toxicity, including, reportedly, thrombophlebitis, skin eruptions, fever, deafness and kidney damage. It is little wonder that methicillin was so warmly welcomed, despite the introduction of an improved version of vancomycin and a better understanding of avoidance of unwanted effects.

The earliest strains of MRSA could be treated with a variety of agents such as erythromycin, chloramphenicol and kanamycin, and later gentamicin, fusidic acid and rifampicin. It was even suggested that a combination of methicillin and kanamycin would be effective. However, as resistance accumulated, and particularly with the advent of EMRSA, vancomycin returned to wide-spread use. Indeed, although it was still an inconvenient antibiotic to use, since it had to be given by intravenous infusion and care was necessary to avoid reactions, it was soon very widely seen as the antibiotic of choice for MRSA infections.[46,50]

Vancomycin 'was difficult to administer, by the intravenous route, causing endophlebitis, and more serious toxicity in the form of eighth nerve damage and nephrotoxicity resulted from (its) use... There can be no place for (it) in modern antibiotic therapy.'

Murdoch (1966)[53]

'Vancomycin is the cornerstone of the therapy of MRSA infection'.

Cookson and Phillips (1990)[22]

The introduction of another glycopeptide, teicoplanin, albeit not in all countries, administrable intramuscularly, widened the choice.[22] Eventually, diminished susceptibility to the glycopeptides began to appear and finally full resistance in rare strains.[55] Fortunately, the pharmaceutical industry developed new antistaphylococcal drugs, and the streptogramin mixture quinupristin-dalfopristin and linezolid, belonging to a new class of antibiotics, the oxazolidinones, eased the situation. Unsurprisingly, reports of resistance soon followed their introduction.[55] These developments are discussed later in this book, as is the now widely recognised need for the development of further new antibiotics, no mean undertaking in view of the expense of their development and licensing.

Lessons from the past

At the very beginning of the period of this review, the Professor of Microbiology at St Thomas's Hospital, Ronald Hare (who had been a junior colleague of Alexander Fleming at St Mary's Hospital, and used to address us, largely about his perceived failings, when we became members of his department at our obligatory daily tea-time gatherings) taught us about the sources, routes and portals of staphylococcal infections in hospitals, based on his own experience. Carriers and infected patients were well recognised as the sources; direct contact, fomites and airborne skin squames (one of his particular interests) the routes; and hospitalised patients (especially, at the time, those with surgical wounds) in contact with these, the ever-ready recipients. Attempts to eradicate carriage were made (including Elek's maverick approach which may yet have lessons for us), means of limiting contact and the access of airborne spread were fully applied, and attempts to protect the susceptible, notably by the use of prophylactic antibiotics, and the introduction of plenum ventilation in operating theatres, were widely applied. All this lead to an increasing appreciation of the diversity of staphylococcal strains, and of their adaptation to their environment.

As for resistant staphylococci, Mary Barber had applied her law of prevention of the emergence of resistance at the Hammersmith Hospital and at St Thomas's Hospital (in Ronald Hare's department, where two strong personalities made for some discomfort) by promoting the control of cross-infection and of antibiotic use. No new principles were developed for the control of MRSA when they appeared.

Although the tools available to us may have improved, we can add little to the principles. However, because of the gap years of the late 1960s and the early 1970s when staphylococci generally caused fewer problems, many of the new generation who had to deal with EMRSA had little knowledge of the earlier work on staphylococci and often seemed intent on re-inventing the wheel. Even now, it would be far from a waste of time to read the early papers from the pioneers.

But, a note of caution. All we have learned has not taught us how to prevent the march of antibiotic resistance in general, or of methicillin resistance in particular, on a demographic scale.

Conclusions

MRSA have now been with us for over 40 years, ever since methicillin became available as a means of detecting them. They were initially rare, and even now their distribution is patchy, with some parts of the world currently reporting few isolates while others report them in very large numbers. It has been necessary to make major surveillance efforts to detect the extent of the problem, and to introduce expensive measures to prevent and control outbreaks. Therapeutic options dwindled during a period when no new antibiotic classes were produced, and vancomycin and teicoplanin became drugs of first and last choice. When resistance to these glycopeptides was reported, the situation seemed desperate, but quinupristin-dalfopristin and linezolid promised relief. The development of resistance to each in turn suggested that reliance on them in the longer term might be unwise.

Unless and until the pandemic subsides – and one hopes that it might follow the probably spontaneous fate of the multiresistant 'Hospital Staphylococcus' of the 1950s and 1960s – there is a need for continuing surveillance, the application of effective control measures, and the development of novel antibacterial agents, perhaps including vaccines. At the same time, a radically fresh scientific approach to the control of MRSA might be encouraged.

References

1. McDonald PJ. Methicillin-resistant staphylococci. *Med J Aust* 1982; **i**: 445–6.

2. Kirby WMM. Treatment of generalized staphylococcal infections. *Postgrad Med J* 1964; **40 (Suppl)**: 37–9.

3. Batchelor FR, Doyle FP, Nayler JHC, Rolinson GN. Synthesis of penicillin 6-aminopenicillanic acid in penicillin fermentations. *Nature* 1959; **183**: 257–8.

4. Rolinson GN. Forty years of β-lactam research. *J Antimicrob Chemother* 1998; **41**: 589–603.

5. Knox R. A new penicillin (BRL 1214) active against penicillin-resistant staphylococci. *BMJ* 1960; **ii**: 690–3.

6. Thompson REM, Whitby JL, Harding JW. Treatment of experimental penicillin-resistant staphylococcal lesions with BRL 1241. *BMJ* 1960; **ii**: 706–8.

7. Douthwaite AH, Trafford JAP. A new synthetic penicillin. *BMJ* 1960; **ii**: 687–90.

8. Stewart GT, Nixon HH, Coles HMT. Report on clinical use of BRL 1241. *BMJ* 1960; **ii**: 703–6.

9. Brumfitt W, Williams JD. (eds) *Therapy with the new penicillins. Postgrad Med J* 1964; **40 (Suppl)**: 1–214.

10. Barber M. Methicillin-resistant staphylococci. *J Clin Pathol* 1961; **14**: 385–93.

11. Elek SD, Fleming PC. A new technique for the control of hospital cross-infection. *Lancet* 1960; **ii**: 569–72.

12. Goldfarb S, James GCW. Abolition of staphylococcal cross-infection in a surgical ward. *BMJ* 1963; **i**: 305–8.

13. Stewart GT, Holt RJ. Evolution of natural resistance to the newer penicillins. *BMJ* 1963; **i**: 308–11.

14. Rolinson GN, Batchelor, FR, Stevens S, Wood JC, Chain E. Bacteriological studies on a new penicillin – BRL 1241. *Lancet* 1960; **ii**: 564–7.

15. Jevons MP. 'Celbenin'-resistant staphylococci. *BMJ* 1961; **i**: 124–5.

16. Rolinson GN. 'Celbenin'-resistant staphylococci. *BMJ* 1961; **i**: 125–6.

17. Knox R. 'Celbenin'-resistant staphylococci. *BMJ* 1961; **i**: 126.

18. Barber M. Methicillin-resistant staphylococci and hospital infection. *Postgrad Med J* 1964; **40 (Suppl)**: 178–81.

19. Parker MT. Jevons MP. A survey of methicillin resistance in *Staphylococcus aureus*. *Postgrad Med J* 1964; **40 (suppl)**: 170–8.

20. Pal SC, Ghosh BG. Methicillin-resistant staphylococci. *J Ind Med Assoc* 1964; **42**: 512–7.

21. Borowski J, Kamienska K, Rutecka I. Methicillin-resistant staphylococci. *BMJ* 1964; **i**: 983.

22. Cookson B. Phillips I. Methicillin-resistant staphylococci. *J Appl Bacteriol* 1990; **Symposium Suppl**: 55S–70S.

23. Annear DI. The effect of temperature on resistance of *Staphylococcus aureus* to methicillin and some other antibiotics. *Med J Aust* 1968; **i**: 444–6.

24. Chabbert Y-A. Baudens J-G. Souches de staphylocoques resistant naturellement a la méthicilline et a la 5-méthyl-3-phényl-4-oxazolyyl-pénicilline. *Ann Inst Pasteur* 1962; **103**: 222–30.

25. Barber M, Waterworth PM. Antibacterial activity of the penicillins. *BMJ* 1962; **i**: 1159–64.

26. Wenzel RP, Nettleman MD, Jones RN, Pfaller MA. Methicillin-resistant *Staphylococcus aureus*: implications for the 1990s and effective control measures. *Am J Med* 1991; **91 (Suppl 3B)**: 221S–227S.

27. Benner EJ, Kayser FH. Growing clinical significance of methicillin-resistant *Staphylococcus aureus*. *Lancet* 1968; **ii**: 741–4.

28. Rosendahl K. Current national patterns. In: Brachman PS, Eickhoff TC. (eds) *Proceedings of the International Conference on Nosocomial Infections*. Chicago, IL: American Hospitals Association, 1971; 11–6.

29. Thompson RL, Cabezudo I, Wenzel RP. Epidemiology of nosocomial infections caused by methicillin-resistant *Staphylococcus aureus*. *Ann Intern Med* 1982; **97**: 309–17.

30. Barber M. Whitehead JEM. Bacteriophage types in penicillin-resistant staphylococcal infection. *BMJ* 1949; **ii**: 565–9.

31. Jevons MP, Parker MT. The evolution of new hospital strains of *Staphylococcus aureus*. *J Clin Pathol* 1964; **17**: 243–50.

32. Brown DFJ, Reynolds PE. Intrinsic resistance to β-lactam antibiotics in *Staphylococcus aureus*. *FEBS Lett* 1980; **122**: 275–8.

33. Hartman BJ, Tomasz A. Low-affinity penicillin-binding protein associated with β-lactam resistance in *Staphylococcu aureus*. *J Bacteriol* 1984; **158**: 513–6.

34. Murakami K. Tomasz A. Involvement of multiple genetic determinants in high-level methicillin resistance in *Staphylococcus aureus*. *J Bacteriol* 1989; **171**: 874–9.

35. Skurray R in précis of discussions and comments to Marples and Cooke (see reference 43).

36. Rountree PM, Beard MA. Hospital strains of *Staphylococcus aureus* with particular reference to methicillin-resistant strains. *Med J Aust* 1968; **ii**: 1163–5.

37. Pavillard R, Harvey K. Douglas D *et al*. Epidemic of hospital-acquired infection due to methicillin-resistant *Staphylococcus aureus* in major Victorian hospitals. *Med J Aust* 1982; **i**: 451–4.

38. Gilbert GL, Asche V, Hewstone AS, Mathieson JL. Methicillin-resistant *Staphylococcus aureus* in neonatal nurseries. *Med J Aust* 1982; **i**: 455–9.

39. Brumfitt W, Hamilton-Miller J. Methicillin-resistant *Staphylococcus aureus*. *N Engl J Med* 1989; **320**: 1188–96.

40. Duckworth G, Lothian JLE, Williams JD. Methicillin-resistant *Staphylococcus aureus*: report of an outbreak in a London teaching hospital. *J Hosp Infect* 1988; **11**: 1–15.

41. Townsend DE, Ashdown N, Bolton S *et al*. The international spread of methicillin-resistant *Staphylococcus aureus*. *J Hosp Infect* 1987; **9**: 60–71.

42. Phillips I. Epidemic potential and pathogenicity in outbreaks of infection with MRSA and EMREC. *J Hosp Infect* 1991; **18 (Suppl A)**: 197–201.

43. Marples RR, Cooke EM. Current problems with methicillin-resistant *Staphylococcus aureus*. *J Hosp Infect* 1988; **11**: 381–92.

44. Lacey RW. Multi-resistant *Staphylococcus aureus* – a suitable case for inactivity. *J Hosp Infect* 1987; **9**: 103–5.

45. EARSS European Antimicrobial Resistance Surveillance System 2000. National Institute of Public health and the Environment, The Netherlands. <www.earss.rivm.nl>.

46. Mulligan ME, Murray-Leisure KA, Ribner BS *et al*. Methicillin-resistant *Staphylococcus aureus*: a consensus review of the microbiology, pathogenesis, and epidemiology with implications for prevention and management. *Am J Med* 1993; **94**: 313–28.

47. Cookson B, Peters B, Webster M *et al*. Staff carriage of epidemic methicillin-resistant *Staphylococcus aureus*. *J Clin Microbiol* 1989; **27**: 1471–6.

48. Cookson B, Phillips I. Epidemic methicillin-resistant *Staphylococcus aureus*. *J Antimicrob Chemother* 1988; **24 (Suppl C)**: 57–65.

49. Allison D, Galloway A. Guidelines for the control of epidemic methicillin-resistant *Staphylococcus aureus*. *J Hosp Infect* 1986; **7**: 193–201.

50. Working Party of the Hospital Infection Society and British Society for Antimicrobial Chemotherapy. Revised guidelines for the control of epidemic methicillin-resistant *Staphylococcus aureus*. *J Hosp Infect* 1990; **16**: 351–77.

51. Working Party of the British Society for Antimicrobial Chemotherapy and the Hospital Infection Society. Guidelines on the control of methicillin-resistant *Staphylococcus aureus* in the community. *J Hosp Infect* 1995; **31**: 1–12.

52. Gillet Y, Issartel B, Vanhems P *et al*. Association between strains carrying gene for Panton-Valentine leucocidin and highly lethal necrotizing pneumonia in young immunocompetent patients. *Lancet* 2002; **359**: 753–9.

53. Murdoch JMcC. Dangers of antibiotic therapy. In Ridley M, Phillips I. (eds) *The therapeutic use of antibiotics in hospital practice*. Edinburgh: Livingstone, 1966; 81.

54. Chambers HF. Methicillin-resistant staphylococci. *Clin Microbiol Rev* 1988; **1**: 173–86.

55. Woodford N. Biological counterstrike: antibiotic resistance mechanisms of Gram-positive cocci. *Clin Microbiol Infect* 2005; **11 (Suppl 3)**: 2–21.

Further reading

For further useful citations see the review papers given as references 22, 26, 39, 46, 54, 55 and those following the introductory paper of McDonald (reference 1).

2. Pathogenesis and immunology of MSSA and MRSA carriage and infection

Alex van Belkum

Infectious syndromes caused by
S. aureus
Virulence factors of S. aureus
Innate immune evasion
Humoral immunity
Cellular immunity
Mucosal colonisation and local
inflammatory responses
Interference therapy, passive
immunotherapy and vaccines
Are MRSA more virulent or invoking
different immune responses than
MSSA?
Conclusions

Infectious syndromes caused by Staphylococcus aureus

Staphylococcus aureus persistently colonises at least one-third of mankind. It does so in the nasopharynx, the gut, groin and all other physiological niches which are warm and humid. The interaction between man and microbe is usually considered neutral. There is no documentation of obvious positive or detrimental influences exerted by the resident bacteria while being in the colonising rather than the infectious state. However, we seem to be walking on the edge: once our physical and immunological defences wane, *S. aureus* may seize the opportunity and cause infections. These range from self-limiting gastro-enteritis to highly invasive and life-threatening bacteraemia and sepsis. This implies that the pathology and immunology of the interactions between bacteria and man is complex and that the various forms of co-existence require different and well-regulated host–microbe interactions. Antigenic diversity, availability of receptors and ligands, secretion of toxins or other virulence factors, physical barriers, the innate immune components and the development of an acquired, more specific immune response by the host, all contribute to the final outcome – balanced colonisation or (ir)reversible infection.

The clinical importance of *S. aureus* infections became even more relevant upon the emergence of its methicillin-resistant variants (MRSA). Over the past 50 years, MRSA has gained in prevalence as an important nosocomial pathogen and it still has an important impact on hospital-acquired infection rates, although prevalence does vary across Europe. Recent inventories revealed that the incidence of *S. aureus* bloodstream infections per 100,000 inhabitants can vary from, for instance, 23, 25, 27 to 32 when considering Iceland, Austria, Denmark and Ireland, respectively. Interestingly, the associated MRSA incidence is 0%, 15%, less than 1% and 42%. Such differences can usually be explained by variation in local antibiotic policies or hospital infection control measures (or a combination of the both). These data do not reveal whether or not MRSA is a more successful pathogen than methicillin-susceptible *S. aureus* (MSSA). Precise definition of the latter is a highly complex issue.

The purpose of this chapter is to sketch *S. aureus* virulence potential and its associated host responses. Essentially, and in the apparent absence of data proving the opposite, MRSA and MSSA will be considered equal.

> The acquisition of antibiotic resistance does not immediately imply the availability of different pathogenic traits and, consequently, is not definitely associated with a higher invasive disease potential.

Whether this is true will be discussed at the end of the chapter by questioning whether clonal divergence or, alternatively, the random distribution of accessory genes is basic to differences in virulence between MRSA and MSSA. It must be emphasised that this chapter will not be complete but an effort has been made to at least cover the most important virulence factors and immunological features of S. aureus colonisation and infection.

Virulence factors of S. aureus

S. aureus is equipped with a multitude of so-called virulence factors. A virulence factor is defined as a bacterial entity which is able to exert a detrimental effect on a host organism. Virulence factors can be superficially stratified into soluble and cell-wall-bound ones. These can each be further stratified into protein and (lipidated, amidated or otherwise modified) oligo- and polysaccharides. The soluble category primarily is constituted by toxins and a variety of exo-enzymes. These are usually involved in the preparation of the host epithelial cell matrix for bacterial attachment or persistence. Toxins may also have a 'bacterial food-oriented' function. The cell-wall attached compounds are frequently involved in physical anchoring of the bacterial cell to the host matrix. Concomitantly, major cell wall structures and the well-exposed anchors are the target of host immune responses. Many of the bacterial virulence and adherence factors are co-regulated through concerted genetic networks. Networks guiding virulence gene expression at the molecular level are, among others, the accessory gene regulator (Agr) and the staphylococcal accessory gene regulator (Sar) systems. These well-conserved molecular switches facilitate the expression of specific groups of genes at certain stages of the microbial life cycle. It must be emphasised that the current improvements in the technology suited for visualising the protein complement (proteomics) or complete polysaccharides content (glycomics) of a cell are continuously expanding the number of characterised S. aureus virulence factors.

Polysaccharides and other non-proteinaceous macromolecules

Peptidoglycan (PG) is one of the most abundant cell wall constituent of S. aureus. It is built from alternating N-acetylglucosamine and N-acetylmuraminic acid units, the polymers of which are cross linked by pentaglycine bridges. The main function of the PG complex is to maintain cellular structure: it provides a rigid envelope for the cell contents. PG has endotoxic properties, is implicated in chronic inflammation and it can cause organ dysfunctioning in experimental animals. Wall teichoic acids (WTAs) are embedded in the PG matrix and also constitute an important fraction of the bacterial cell wall. WTAs have been identified as components that are important in establishing nasal colonisation. WTAs are not highly inflammatory components of the staphylococcal surface, although several studies suggest that these compounds contribute to the severity of staphylococcal sepsis.

S. aureus produces a slimy, capsular polysaccharide and two major forms can be distinguished using serological tests – types 5 and 8. These are both built of repeated trisaccharides consisting of N-acetyl mannosaminuronic acid, N-acetyl-L-fucosamine and N-acetyl-D-fucosamine. Interestingly, capsular type 5 is associated with increased virulence and decreased opsonophagocytosis and neutrophil-mediated killing.

Peptides and proteins

Usually, microbial surface components recognising adhesive matrix molecules (MSCRAMMs) are staphylococcal proteins constituting the prime determinants of bacterial adhesion to host compounds. A variety of such proteins, covalently attached to the cell wall through an LPXTG amino acid motif, are able to bind a wide spectrum of host molecules. Such molecules include immunoglobulins, keratins, fibrinogen, fibronectin, collagen and many others. The specificity of the reactions allows for precise and tissue-specific attachment of S. aureus to host-cells. It is interesting to note that many physically and functionally different MSCRAMMs exist. Protein A, for instance, binds the Fcγ domain of antibodies. Protein A also recognises the tumour necrosis factor-α (TNF-α) receptor 1, leading to more severe presentation of staphylococcal pneumonia. MSCRAMMs fulfil a broad spectrum of functions, most of which are associated with (maintaining) residence in certain ecological niches. Obviously, these multifunctional proteins affect staphylococcal virulence potential.

Various proteins with different structure and function are secreted by the bacterium. These include coagulase, extracellular fibrinogen binding protein, the extracellular matrix protein or the extracellular adherence protein. The extra-cellular adherence protein (Eap), for instance, interferes with wound healing by dis-balancing host repair and immunological defence mechanisms.

S. aureus produces a diversity of exoproteins and cytotoxins. Most, if not all, strains produce α-, β-, γ-, and δ-hemolysins, nucleases, proteases, lipases, hyaluronidase and collagenase. Hemolysins are porins that help lyse a variety of host cells. Various cytokines are induced and several cell types are attracted at sites of hemolysin production. In addition, some strains produce the toxic shock syndrome toxin-1 (TSST-1), one or more enterotoxins (A-E, G-I, the number is still expanding), the exfoliative toxin A or B and leukocidins. The hemolysins and the leukocidins inhibit the immune response, TSST-1 and the enterotoxins represent the pyrogenic toxin superantigens (PTSAgs). These compounds are intermediately sized proteins (20–30 kDa) with significant primary structure homology but

significant structural diversity. A very interesting porin is the Panton-Valentine leukocidin, which is structurally similar to the α-toxin. PVL is a secreted toxin that forms its pores most probably in the mitochondrial outer membrane. PVL kills peripheral mononuclear cells in vitro, either by necrosis or apoptosis depending on the PVL concentration.

PTSAgs derail the immune response and, in the case of S. aureus, are usually encoded by accessory genetic elements such as plasmids, bacteriophages or pathogenicity islands. Nineteen different PTSAgs have been described to date, a number that is still expanding. PTSAgs bypass the conventional antigen recognition route by directly cross-linking major histocompatibility complex II (MHCII) molecules on antigen-presenting cells with T-cell receptors. This leads to activation of large T-cell populations and cytokine release. This again may result in toxic shock syndrome and possibly septic shock. Enterotoxin A, for instance, is associated with elevated virulence potential of the strain involved. Staphylococcal enterotoxins D and J display similar activities. TSST-I is by far the best known staphylococcal superantigen. It is causative in tampon-associated disease in women and neonatal toxic shock syndrome-like exanthematous disease. It affects Vβ2+ T-cell proliferation and the expression of CD45RO. Antibodies against TSST-I suppress T-cell activation and protects against development of disease.

Innate immune evasion

S. aureus has developed many different strategies for the evasion of human innate immune responses. For instance, S. aureus is able to degrade certain antimicrobial peptides specifically. Cathelicidin, one of the most important antistaphylococcal defensins, can be inactivated by aureolysin, an S. aureus specific metalloprotease. Proteolytic degradation of defensins contributes to resistance of S. aureus to the innate immune response. Modification of WTAs renders a cell more resistant to defensin-mediated killing as well.

To survive in the intracellular compartment of phagocytes, *S. aureus* has two superoxide dismutase genes at its disposal. The enzyme destroys reactive oxygen as does catalase, a protein shared by all *S. aureus* strains. Carotenoid pigments provide a third class of anti-peroxide compounds. Interference with complement is another very popular theme among staphylococci and this is addressed in a variety of ways. The extracellular fibrinogen binding protein Efb blocks classical pathway-dependent opsonisation. The extracellular adherence protein inhibits leukocyte chemotaxis. A protein called chemotaxis inhibiting protein (CHIPS) impairs the response of neutrophils and monocytes to formylated peptides and complement proteins. CHIPS binds to the formyl peptide receptor and the complement factor 5a receptor, thereby interfering at multiple stages of the complement activation pathways.

Humoral immunity

Antistaphylococcal antibodies can be detected in essentially all human beings. The antibody levels tend to rise upon infection but, in general, the antibody levels are too low to be protective. There is no obvious secondary response upon re-infection and immune memory seems to be limited. Lack of antibodies to PTSAg is predictive of susceptibility to toxic shock syndrome of the host. Antibodies against MSCRAMMs protect against *in vitro* bacterial adherence to the immobilised ligand of such MSCRAMMs.

> No generalised scheme of antibody induction in people infected with, or simply carrying, *S. aureus* can be proposed.

Cellular immunity

For many years, it has been assumed that the antibody-mediated response to *S. aureus* was the major, maybe even the only, host reaction upon infection. However, it has been demonstrated that superantigens do induce a significant T-cell response as well. These interactions stimulate cytokine production. Cytokines are proteins that are produced by white blood cells and others after induction by pathogens. There is enormous variation in the nature and effects of these human cytokines. Overall, these cytokines initiate important immunological cascades aimed at the suppression of infection. Major effects are the activation of T cells, the induction of inflammatory mediators, terminal differentiation of B cells, and the enhancement of immunoglobulin secretion by B cells. The cytokine-induced response is geared towards a generalised activation of basic immune disposition. The cellular immunology of *S. aureus* colonisation and infection is still an underexplored research area and still much remains to be gained, both from the scientific and the clinical perspective.

Mucosal colonisation and local inflammatory responses

In the presence of *S. aureus* cells, the epithelial production of host defensins is up-regulated. This results in a sort of persistent inflammatory state during staphylococcal colonisation. Nasal fluid from *S. aureus* carriers is defective in killing endogenous *S. aureus* cells and other nasal carriage isolates. Laboratory strains may still be effectively killed, however. The nasal secretions are not defective in lactoferrin or lysozyme.

Microbes need means to hide in the usually hostile host environment. This may be achieved by assuming a life-style that is different from the usual planktonic one. Many organisms grow in highly organised systems called biofilms. It is currently not clear whether biofilm formation is important in the *S. aureus* life cycle or for establishing nasal colonisation. Biofilms may be important to *S. aureus* in order to survive in, or on, the human body; for instance, while initiating or maintaining nasal colonisation. The formation of staphylococcal biofilms is an important issue since it is thought to confer lowered antimicrobial susceptibility levels and immune resistance as well.

> It is currently unknown whether MRSA show an enhanced propensity towards the development of biofilms as compared to MSSA. It is not even known whether biofilm formation is a variable parameter among MSSA.

Interference therapy, passive immunotherapy and vaccines

Colonisation by MSSA or MRSA can be approached from an ecological perspective. Colonisation that gives rise to clinically relevant infections needs to be resolved and this can, possibly, be done by local microbial interference, either with non-staphylococcal species or with non-virulent or non-antibiotic resistant strains of *S. aureus*. Experimental proof of the relevance of the interaction between MSSA and MRSA in the anterior nares was recently generated by longitudinal follow-up of the MRSA/MSSA colonisation state of patients at re-admission to hospital. MRSA alone was carried by 8% of the patients, 17% carried MSSA alone, 0.6% carried both MRSA and MSSA, the remainder (74.3%) did not carry staphylococci at all. The fraction of 'mixed carriers' was small which suggested that competition for the nasal niche is taking place. Recent studies involving artificial inoculation of volunteers with mixtures of different *S. aureus* strains demonstrated that mixtures do not persevere: within a period of weeks, strains either disappeared altogether or a single 'survivor' occupied the vestibulum nasi. Other bacterial species such as *Lactobacillus fermentum*, *Corynebacterium* spp. or several coagulase-negative staphylococci are able to compete for space with *S. aureus*. The mode of interference between isolates of a species can be considered a virulence factor, especially if the more virulent bacteria are able to out-compete the less virulent ones.

Passive immunisation with human plasma-derived anti-*S. aureus* immunoglobulins was tested in pneumonia models in mice. Both nasally and systemically administered antibodies prevented infection. Tefibazumab is a humanised monoclonal antibody with high affinity for ClfA. The monoclonal was protective in a mouse sepsis model and further human studies are now in progress. Recent studies showed that it is well tolerated and can be administered to reach high levels in the circulation. No antibodies against the monoclonal were induced in healthy volunteers.

Various staphylococcal antigens have been used for active immunisation. In the case of bovine mastitis, a trial involving a trivalent capsular vaccine (serotypes 5, 8 and 336) showed clear antibody response in vaccinated animals. Whether this is protective to infection is currently not clear. Capsules of serotypes 5 and 8, immobilised onto genetically detoxified recombinant exoprotein A from *Pseudomonas aeruginosa*, have been shown to elicit a strong bactericidal immune response in end-stage renal disease patients. The human equivalent of the capsular vaccine, StaphVAX™, only contains capsular polysaccharides of types 5 and 8 coupled to an immune-stimulating carrier protein but clinical trials have been disappointing.

> Alternative therapies for staphylococcal infections are urgently required.

Are MRSA more virulent or invoking different immune responses than MSSA?

Overall differences in virulence between strains of *S. aureus* are best expressed as differences in virulence gene potential between such strains. It is interesting to note that MRSA are usually highly transmissible and it has been suggested that MRSA carriage more frequently results in infection than MSSA carriage does. However, MRSA carriage is primarily nosocomially derived, suggesting that especially those that are already ill get colonised. This influences the chances of developing a staphylococcal infection, of course. Recent Dutch studies have shown that *S. aureus* carriage as such may protect from mortality in case of a staphylococcal bacteraemia. A recent study on ventilator-associated pneumonia once more underscored how difficult comparative MRSA/MSSA pathogenicity studies are: the authors found that differences in patient characteristics, initial intensive care treatment and time of residence in the intensive care units were strongly confounding factors. This led them to conclude that, in the case of ventilator-associated pneumonia, no excess death due to MRSA infection could be documented.

MRSA and MSSA are not essentially different from a genetic point of view.

> The emergence of MRSA from locally circulating MSSA is not a frequent event and universal spread of a few successful clones seems to be the more frequent scenario.

This implies that the epidemic MRSA clones are optimally adapted to humans and this may suggest that successful MRSA should not be highly pathogenic. It has been documented that strains of *S. aureus* expressing capsular type 5 are more virulent than strains expressing a type 8 capsule.

Is MRSA disease generally more serious? In case of the PVL-positive (usually community acquired) MRSA this clearly seems to be the case. Interestingly, PVL seems to be confined to MRSA harbouring type IV or type V staphylococcal cassette chromosome (SCCmec) elements, belonging to one or a limited number of staphylococcal lineages. Horizontal gene transfer must have been involved at some stage. However, most, if not all, PVL-positive MSSA also derive from deep-seated infections. Apparently, PVL does contribute to disease severity but does so for both MRSA and MSSA.

The overall difference in virulence between MRSA and MSSA is hard to establish *per se*.

Efforts have been made, however. By comparing Korean patients suffering from endocarditis caused by either MRSA or MSSA, it appeared that persistent bacteraemia was significantly more present among MRSA patients. This resulted in a higher mortality trend too and the authors proposed more aggressive, MRSA-geared antimicrobial treatment in cases of persisting bacteraemia. These findings were biased: co-morbidity percentages in the MRSA group were much higher, as was nosocomial infection, prior antibiotic usage and mechanical ventilation. A recent, large German study involving 274 intensive care units, 505,487 ICU patients, 6888 cases of nosocomial pneumonia and 2357 cases of primary bloodstream infection failed to deliver a definite answer due to lack of power. The number of studies that document the lack of increased virulence among MRSA is increasing, but so are studies that conclude the opposite. Interestingly, many other features of the MRSA versus MSSA virulence controversy have not yet been investigated.

It is well established that patients infected with MRSA are usually prone to prolonged hospitalisation incurring doubling of the overall costs as compared to MSSA-infected patients. Would the resistance trait by itself contribute to enhanced microbial virulence? This could be the case but another simple explanation for the observed differences in attributed mortality and morbidity could be that therapy fails more frequently, particularly in the case of the severely weakened patients. In such cases, the observed 'virulence' is due to a lack of treatment options rather than bacterial virulence potential.

Conclusions

Both MRSA and MSSA are able to colonise the human body. This does not seem to be pathogenic to a healthy person. The immune response evoked during colonisation is still enigmatic. Locally, a mild inflammatory response is observed and systemic antibodies will be generated. It is not known what are the main staphylococcal immunogens and the cellular response invoked is also still unclear. When infection develops, enhanced antibody responses are observed, but the kinetics and dynamics of this process are still poorly understood. During infection, innate and acquired immune responses help fight the invading micro-organisms which, in turn, develop various mechanisms that help cope with host defence. The interactions between host and microbe, both during colonisation and infection, are slowly being unravelled but we are certainly not at the stage where we can distinguish between MRSA- and MSSA-specific pathogenic or immunogenic stimuli.

Further reading

Dall'Antonia M, Coen PG, Wilks M, Whiley A, Millar M. Competition between methicillin-sensitive and –resistant *Staphylococcus aureus* in the anterior nares. *J Hosp Infect* 2005; **61**: 62–7.

Dinges MM, Orwin PM, Schleivert PM. Exotoxins of *Staphylococcus aureus*. *Clin Microbiol Rev* 2000; **13**: 16–34.

Dryla A, Prustomersky S, Gelbmann D *et al.* Comparison of antibody repertoires against *Staphylococcus aureus* in healthy individuals and in acutely infected patients. *Clin Diagn Lab Immunol* 2005; **12**: 387–98.

Foster TJ. Immune evasion by staphylococci. *Nat Rev Microbiol* 2005; **3**: 948–58.

Fournier B, Philpott DJ. Recognition of *Staphylococcus aureus* by the innate immune system. *Clin Microbiol Rev* 2005; **18**: 521–40.

Gastmeier P, Sohr D, Geffers C, Behnke M, Daschner F, Ruden H. Mortality risk factors with nosocomial *Staphylococcus aureus* infections in intensive care units: results from the German nosocomial infection surveillance system (KISS). *Infection* 2005; **33**: 50–5.

Genestier AL, Michallet MC, Prevost G *et al.* *Staphylococcus aureus* Panton-Valentine leukocidin directly targets mitochondria and induces Bax-independent apoptosis of human neutrophils. *J Clin Invest* 2005; **115**: 3117–27.

Holtfreter S, Broker BM. Staphylococcal antigens: do they play a role in sepsis? *Arch Immunol Ther Exp* 2005; **53**: 13–27.

Rooijakkers SHM, Van Kessel KPM, Van Strijp JAG. Staphylococcal innate immune evasion. *Trends Microbiol* 2006; In press.

Shinefield H, Black S, Fattom A *et al.* Use of a *Staphylococcus aureus* conjugate vaccine in patients receiving hemodialysis. *N Engl J Med* 2002; **346**: 491–6.

Visser L, De Heer HJ, Boven LA *et al.* Proinflammatory bacterial PG as a cofactor for the development of central nervous system autoimmune disease. *J Immunol* 2005; **174**: 808–16.

Yoon HJ, Choi JY, Kim CO, Kim JM, Song YG. A comparison of clinical features and mortality among methicillin-resistant and methicillin-sensitive strains of *Staphylococcus aureus* endocarditis. *Yonsei Med J* 2005; **46**: 496–502.

3. The evolution of MRSA

Ben RD Short, Mark C Enright

Early MRSA
Investigating the evolution of MRSA
Evolutionary mechanisms
Evolutionary history of MRSA
Concluding remarks

The first MRSA were isolated in the UK more than 40 years ago. Although this strain (or clone) rapidly spread to different continents it seemingly lacked the ability inherent in modern MRSA, to cause large outbreaks and to become endemic in hospital settings. Some advances in modern medicine have led to our increasing reliance on antibiotics and immunosuppressive agents, and routine use of in-dwelling vascular devices, all of which promote colonisation and invasion of the host by pathogenic bacteria that can adapt to thrive in the hospital environment. In this chapter, we outline our current knowledge of how *Staphylococcus aureus* established itself as the most important hospital-acquired pathogen world-wide and describe the features that allow it to adapt rapidly to novel niches – expanding its host range to healthy individuals outside of healthcare settings.

Early MRSA

S. aureus has always maintained a close relationship with humans. The organism is carried in 30–40% of the population across all age classes, living in the anterior nares from where it is frequently shed onto the skin. The organism causes mainly minor skin infections such as pimples and boils and only very rarely does it invade sterile tissues. Despite this low 'attack rate', its ubiquity in human populations makes it a major cause of community-acquired sepsis.

> Prior to the introduction of antibiotics, *S. aureus* sepsis resulted in death in > 80% of patients in one long-term study in a Boston hospital.

Penicillin drastically reduced this mortality although, within 2 years of its introduction, resistant isolates had been identified. These isolates carry a plasmid-borne β-lactamase enzyme that can hydrolyse the antibiotic. The β-lactamase resistant antibiotic methicillin was introduced in 1959 to combat such isolates and this selected for the emergence of the first MRSA isolate some 2 years later. Methicillin and its modern-day replacements (nafcillin, oxacillin and flucloxacillin) inhibit cell-wall synthesis by binding to proteins involved in cell-wall synthesis – the penicillin binding proteins (PBPs). MRSA have a novel PBP gene that allows cell-wall synthesis to continue in the presence of the antibiotic due to a poor affinity of the PBP protein for β-lactams. This gene, *mecA* is common in the closely related ubiquitous skin commensal *Staphylococcus epidermidis* from where it is thought to have transferred into *S. aureus*.

The first MRSA spread rapidly to become a problem in countries as far afield as Denmark, Uganda and Australia in the 1960s reaching the US in the 1970s. This MRSA clone was only resistant to β-lactam antibiotics and, in the UK and elsewhere, was quite rare and widely regarded as more of a nuisance than the serious public health threat we perceive today. Up until the early 1990s, MRSA were responsible for 1–2% of *S. aureus* bacteraemia in the UK; however, this dramatically increased to > 45% at the end of that decade – a rapid increase mirrored in many industrialised countries. How did this epidemic happen?

Investigating the evolution of MRSA

It is clear that modern MRSA are very different to those seen in the 1960s – they are frequently multidrug resistant and can spread very quickly causing large outbreaks. Modern MRSA also seem to be able to persist in clinical settings and have become endemic in most UK hospitals. So where did these modern MRSA come from? An early theory proposed that *mecA* was acquired only once by the *S. aureus* and that all MRSA were descendants of this one cell. The methods developed to disprove this theory and their subsequent application to large samples of isolates from around the world have given us a much better understanding of how MRSA first evolved and the origins of modern isolates.

The ability to discriminate, accurately and reliably, between isolates of a bacterial pathogen is crucial in investigating their spread at the local, especially the hospital, level. Outbreaks of MRSA are caused by the rapid dispersal of a single isolate from an index case over a short time scale so that all index-associated infections will be caused by genetically identical (or near-identical) isolates. Conversely, when looking at the global epidemiology of MRSA, this level of discrimination in inappropriate. Two isolates that diverged from a common ancestor can be noticeably different after 40 years of evolutionary change so that, for example, even if a modern MRSA isolate found in the US had descended from the first MRSA seen in England in 1961, so many genetic differences would have accumulated that this relationship would be obscure. Comparison of members of a bacterial species, strain typing, has been used extensively in outbreak situations to trace paths of infection. The most commonly used method, analysis of antibiotic resistance patterns, is used in clinical microbiology laboratories world-wide and this is often useful in early detection of new outbreaks. However, on a background of endemic MRSA in a hospital, outbreaks due to similar strains cannot be resolved by this method and genetically distinct isolates may share common resistance patterns – this is especially true of multiply-antibiotic resistant MRSA clones.

Pulsed-field gel electrophoresis (PFGE)

The application of DNA-based methods (genotyping/DNA fingerprinting) have greatly advanced our understanding of how bacterial pathogens spread. PFGE has emerged to become the most commonly used genotyping method for MRSA outbreak analysis and this technique was for many years the gold standard typing method for *S. aureus*. PFGE is a simple technique based on RFLP (restriction fragment length polymorphism) banding patterns on agarose gels obtained by cleavage of chromosomal DNA by a rare-cutting restriction endonuclease (usually *Sma*I). However, gel patterns vary in quality and are complex in nature making them very difficult to standardise; thus, comparison of patterns between gels and between laboratories is extremely problematic. PFGE is very sensitive to genetic change and observed changes in banding patterns between related isolates are difficult and time-consuming to analyse. Although this method is still the most widely used for short-term epidemiology and local studies, its applicability to evolutionary analyses is limited.

Multilocus sequence typing (MLST)

Access to affordable, high-quality DNA sequencing is now wide-spread among research and diagnostic laboratories and this has seen an increase in the number of studies using sequence-based methods for typing isolates. MLST is now widely used for the unambiguous characterisation of many human pathogens (<http://www.mlst.net>). Sequencing provides an unambiguous strain definition that is easily repeatable and results can be directly compared between laboratories around the world. Also, as we will see later, the data provided are easy to manipulate and analyse *in silico*.

MLST involves the sequencing of internal fragments of (usually) seven genes in the bacterial chromosome that are thought to change slowly with time. Sequencing seven distinct genetic targets also minimises the impact of recent recombinational (DNA exchange) events because the seven genes are widely separated around the genome. Different forms of each of the seven sequences (alleles) are given numbers in databases and these are combined to give a 7-digit allelic profile which can be assigned a sequence type (ST) and compared to other isolates online. On average, 40 alleles are recognised for each of the *S. aureus* MLST targets. The two most common MRSA clones in the UK are known as EMRSA (epidemic MRSA) -15 and -16 and these clones have the allelic profiles 7-6-1-5-8-8-6 and 2-2-2-2-3-3-2, corresponding to sequence types (STs) 22 and 36, respectively. MRSA isolates, their allelic profiles and clinical details from > 20 different countries are currently available on the MLST website and there is an active community of scientists and clinicians involved in tracing the spread of such clones nationally and internationally.

As well as MLST which analyses the 'core genome' of an isolate, information available from genome sequencing of seven strains of *S. aureus* and corresponding microarray information has been used in efforts to understand the processes involved in MRSA evolution (Box 3.1). We also routinely sequence more polymorphic loci such as *spa* and surface exposed (*sas*) genes to further tease out evolutionary relationships.

BURST

BURST (Based Upon Related Sequence Types) is an algorithm devised by Ed Feil at the University of Bath to illustrate the genetic relationships from multilocus datasets provided by techniques such as MLST.

Intended for use on bacteria that exhibit an epidemic population structure (such as *S. aureus*), a dataset of ST numbers and allelic profiles can be entered into the BURST program (<http://www.mlst.net/BURST/burst.htm>) which then groups isolates together into clonal complexes. These clonal complexes are ascertained by grouping together strains that share five out of seven alleles (this stringency can be altered) with at least one other member of the group. The ancestor of each clonal

---

Box 3.1

Genome sequencing and microarray analysis for investigating the evolution of MRSA.

Seven strains of *S. aureus* have had their genomes sequenced including five MRSA isolates, providing an unique abundance of genome data for this species. Having seven genome sequences for this pathogen allows a huge amount of information to be mined using *in silico* comparative genomics and various bioinformatics tools exist for this purpose. Genome sequencing can also turn up novel virulence loci, such as the ACME locus associated with the important community MRSA clone USA300.

In addition to the importance of genome sequencing *per se*, it also allows the production of microarrays, a tool of growing importance for assessing the importance to virulence of different genes.

---

complex should be the genotype which has the largest number of single locus variants (SLVs). BURST has been used to examine *S. aureus* population biology and has proven highly useful in visualising large datasets and teasing out relationships that other methods were unable to do. Figure 3.1 shows the *S. aureus* species visualised using BURST.

Evolutionary mechanisms

How to make an MRSA

MRSA strains are formed by the acquisition of *mecA*, carried on a unique mobile genetic element, SCC*mec* (Staphylococcal Chromosomal Cassette *mec*), into a conserved binding site within an unknown open reading frame, *orfX*, close to the origin of replication of the chromosome. SCC*mec* is unlike other mobile genetic elements such as transposons or phage mediated genes; it most closely resembles a pathogenicity island but lacks virulence factors. The term 'antibiotic resistance island' has been suggested.

The SCC*mec* element has been categorised into five major types (although novel types and subtypes are regularly being discovered) termed

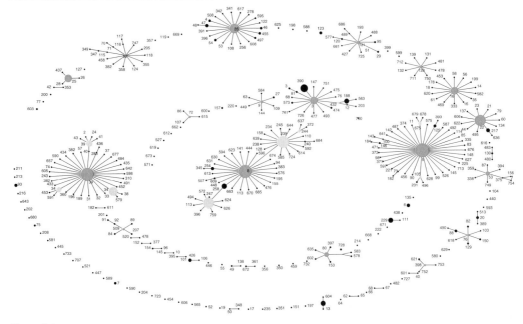

Figure 3.1

Image of *S. aureus* population using BURST. Blue circles represent proposed founder STs of each clonal complex joined to single locus variants by lines. Yellow circles represent proposed sub-group founding STs. The larger the circle the higher the number of isolates in the MLST database of that ST.

I, II, III, and IV and V. All of these types contain the *mecA* gene, which codes for a novel penicillin binding protein, PBP2′. The first MRSA, exemplified by the common laboratory strain COL carries a SCC*mec* I element that only confers resistance to β-lactams. Multiply antibiotic resistant MRSA commonly carry SCC*mec* II or III that confer resistance to other antibiotics such as erythromycin, tetracycline and chloramphenicol although resistance determinants are also found elsewhere in the chromosome. SCC*mec* type IV is the smallest of the elements and the only resistance determinant carried is *mecA* gene. This SCC*mec* element has been shown to be the most promiscuous; one theory is that its small size enables reduces its impact on bacterial fitness when compared to the other larger elements.

The core genome and the importance of 'accessory' genes

Genome sequence and microarray data have been particularly successful in determining an emerging paradigm of bacterial genetics – the distinction between core, conserved genes and more variable, non-essential accessory genes. *In silico* analysis suggests that up to 75% of the *S. aureus* genome may be composed of core genes which include those associated with metabolism and housekeeping functions, common species virulence factors (such as those involved in iron uptake), surface binding proteins and the capsule biosynthetic cluster. The 25% of the genome made up of accessory genes largely contains mobile (or once mobile) genetic elements that can (or have) transfer(ed) horizontally between strains. Many of these genes carry resistance or virulence functions and are carried on bacteriophages, pathogenicity islands, chromosomal cassettes, genomic islands, plasmids and transposons.

Evolutionary history of MRSA

In the early 1990s, it was thought that MRSA arose only once, or at most twice by the single acquisition of the SCC*mec* element by a methicillin susceptible (MSSA) clone. The more recent use of MLST and other molecular typing methods on temporally and geographically diverse isolates suggests a far more dynamic evolutionary history with multiple SCC*mec* acquisitions.

A relatively small number of MRSA clones exist

A diverse range of studies using various typing techniques have shown that *S. aureus* has a largely clonal, epidemic population structure. Using MLST (and BURST analysis) it has been established that there are far fewer clones of successful, hospital MRSA than of MSSA and that these MRSA clones are all descended from one of five unrelated lineages.

This largely clonal population structure is due to a low frequency of recombination (Box 3.2) compared to other more easily transformable species such as *Neisseria meningitidis* and *Streptococcus pneumoniae*. The clonal nature of MRSA populations is reflected not only in studies of core housekeeping genes but also in studies that have looked at far more polymorphic adhesion genes. In fact, an examination of the ratio of synonymous and non-synonymous nucleotide substitutions suggests a strong trend for purifying rather than diversifying selection and this is illustrated in Figure 3.2.

A 'snapshot' study of carried *S. aureus* isolates (including several MRSA isolates) carriage and those found to cause invasive disease in Oxford looked for a link between multilocus genotype

Box 3.2

Recombination versus point mutation in *S. aureus*

MLST is widely used for examining genetic data for a range of pathogens and has been used to estimate how much a bacterial species diversifies by point mutation as opposed to recombination.

Streptococcus pneumoniae, Neisseria meningitidis and *Helicobacter pylori* have been shown to be highly recombigenic and recombination occurs 5–10-fold more in these species than in *S. aureus*. *S. aureus* is not naturally transformable and examination of clonal divergence suggests that point mutation is about 15 times more likely than recombination.

However, phylogenetic analysis suggests that recombination does contribute to the evolution of *S. aureus* over time but not so frequently as to mask the intraspecies phylogenetic signal as has occurred in the previously mentioned species. In fact, two lineages of *S. aureus*, one an important pandemic MRSA lineage, were shown to have been founded by large chromosomal replacements representing up to 20% of the chromosome.

It has been shown that recombination, although rare, is far more likely between closely related strains than between distant phylogenetic lineages. This leads to a model of population structure first proposed by Tibayrenc called 'strict homogamy' which is composed of discrete ecotypes within a species between which there is no (or very little) gene flow.

and virulence and found that no such relationship existed. This suggests that, despite the identification of various virulence factors, strains have a relatively equal ability to cause disease and discounts the notion of hypervirulent clones especially adapted for invading the host. Exceptions to this are strains causing toxinoses such as staphylococcal scalded skin syndrome – caused by exfoliative toxin-producing strains, toxic-shock syndrome and strains expressing toxic-shock syndrome toxin-1 or the enterotoxins B and C, staphylococcal food poisoning caused by enterotoxins A and necrotising pneumonia associated with Panton-Valentine leukocidin.

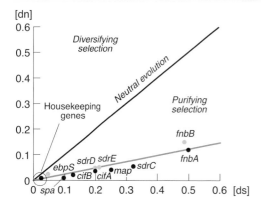

Figure 3.2
Purifying selection. The proportion of synonymous to non-synonymous substitutions was calculated for various *S. aureus* genes. Levels of mutation within housekeeping genes are very low; for the more polymorphic adhesion genes, there is a strong tendency towards purifying selection emphasising the clonal nature of this species.

The first MRSA and acquisition of SCCmec by unrelated clones

Examination of early MRSA isolates from the 1960s using MLST and subsequent BURST analysis showed that nearly all of these isolates belonged to a subgroup of CC8, ST250. All modern isolates of the ST250 subgroup are MRSA, possess SCC*mec* type I, and this clone is considered to have been the original MRSA clone. De Lencastre and colleagues were the first to demonstrated that this first MRSA clone derived from an epidemic methicillin-sensitive *S. aureus* (MSSA) was common in Europe in the 1950s that was also ST250. This strain in itself derived from ST8-MSSA the ancestor of the clonal complex and still a common strain found in carriage and disease.

CC8 represents a very successful and diverse lineage of MRSA; in addition to ST250-MRSA-I, there are three other major pandemic EMRSA STs within CC8 as well as a variety of successful MSSA clones. ST-8 MRSA clones arose from multiple independent acquisitions of SCC*mec* into the successful ST8-MSSA clone and some of these have further diversified to become

modern MRSA, such as the very common and multiply antibiotic resistant Iberian clone.

MRSA has arisen in unrelated lineages due to the multiple acquisition of SCC*mec* and it is thought that the SCC*mec* element was first acquired from a genetically unrelated staphylococcus, possibly *Staphylococcus haemolyticus* (the SCC*mec* element is also found in some other staphylococci including *S. epidermidis*, an important cause of neonatal sepsis and endocarditis). The presence of multiple SCC*mec* types within the same ST indicates that, contrary to previous thought, horizontal transfer of SCC*mec* elements is relatively frequent in *S. aureus*.

Indeed all of the pandemic, ecologically successful, MRSA clones have successful MSSA precursors adapted for effective transmission. A marked example of this are ST5 isolates which are found as successful MSSA from disease or carriage or as epidemic MRSA with each of the four different SCC*mec* types – resistance has thus been acquired at least four times by this MSSA ST alone.

EMRSA-15 and -16 are the predominant MRSA clones currently causing disease in UK hospitals

Greater than 95% of MRSA bacteraemia in the UK is caused by two clones – EMRSA-15 and EMRSA-16 which were first isolated in the early 1990s. MLST and BURST analysis shows that these strains belong to their own CCs – CC22 and CC30, respectively. The complexity of CC22 and CC30 is much less than that found in CC5 or CC8 indicating that these genotypes have emerged relatively recently – they have had little time to accumulate genetic change in contrast to older MRSA clones.

> The greatly increased prevalence of MRSA in the UK is entirely due to the emergence and rapid spread of the EMRSA-15 and EMRSA-16 clones which displaced isolates of EMRSA-3 (ST5) as the most common clone in many hospitals.

Why this should have occurred is unclear as EMRSA-15 is rarely multiply antibiotic resistant in common with EMRSA-3 although EMRSA-15 and EMRSA-16 are though to be more transmissible than previous clones.

The emergence of reduced susceptibility to vancomycin mirrors the emergence of MRSA

With increasing levels of multiply antibiotic-resistant MRSA in many countries, vancomycin has become the most commonly used and trusted agent; it is often referred to as the 'antibiotic of last resort' for treating MRSA infections. Worryingly, since 1997, isolates with reduced susceptibility to this glycopeptide antibiotic (termed VISA – vancomycin intermediate *S. aureus*) have been widely recovered from various locations around the world, although fortunately so far only three VRSA (vancomycin resistant *S. aureus* that possess the *vanA* gene from *Enterococcus faecalis*) strains have been isolated, all in the US. Examples of MRSA with the VISA phenotype have, however, been recovered from every lineage in which MRSA has arisen demonstrating further the adaptability of the species under antibiotic pressure.

This evidence suggests a worrying trend in the evolution of MRSA.

> The multiple independent emergence of vancomycin resistance mirrors the multiple emergence of MRSA from MSSA and could lead to a global increase in the prevalence of VRSA strains.

The impact of this would be exacerbated by the current lack of new antibiotics available in the medium-to-long term that may lead to untreatable MRSA infections in this period.

The rise of community-acquired (CA) MRSA

The evolution of MRSA was, up until the 1990s, largely restricted to the hospital environment where strong selection pressures for antibiotic resistance exist. However, a more recent trend appears to be the increase of MRSA in the community, both as carried isolates, and as those causing aggressive infections in young, otherwise healthy individuals.

A study of CA-MRSA carrying genes for the Panton-Valentine leukocidin (PVL) from around the world found that such isolates could be grouped into six CCs, two of which predominated; strong evidence that CA-MRSA have arisen from diverse genetic backgrounds.

The CA-MRSA MLST type in a particular continent did not correspond to the predominant HA-MRSA type in that area suggesting that CA-MRSA has not simply evolved from successful hospital-acquired clones. This theory is further supported by the fact that CA-MRSA isolates tend to remain susceptible to non-β-lactam antibiotics and contain the smaller type IV SCC*mec* that does not harbour non-β-lactam resistance determinants although some PVL+ multiply antibiotic resistant isolates have recently been discovered.

The PVL toxin genes are expressed by most CA-MRSA and they are associated with a high mortality necrotising pneumonia and, more recently, with cases of necrotising fasciitis. PVL and SCC*mec* IV are widely spaced on the *S. aureus* chromosome and were thus unlikely to have been acquired on the same mobile genetic element. Several studies suggest that CA-MRSA strains harbouring the smaller SCC*mec* IV have an enhanced fitness in comparison with multiresistant hospital-acquired MRSA clones harbouring other SCC*mec* types. It is thought that the decreased metabolic burden associated with having fewer antibiotic resistance determinants could provide a selective advantage in the community setting. Box 3.3 demonstrates the plasticity and adaptability of *S. aureus,* highlighting the ability of successful MSSA clones to become MRSA clones.

Concluding remarks

Despite increasing research efforts aimed at studying the evolution of MRSA there are still

Box 3.3

Re-emergence of early pandemic *S. aureus* as CA-MRSA. During the 1950s, a notorious penicillin-resistant, PVL-expressing *S. aureus* clone emerged (termed 80/81 after its phage lysis pattern) and caused severe hospital and community infections around the world. This clone was largely eliminated by the introduction of methicillin and other β-lactams in the 1960 but has re-emerged after acquiring SCC*mec* IV as an important CA-MRSA clone.

This PVL-containing lineage shares a common ancestor with the important HA-MRSA-16 clone.

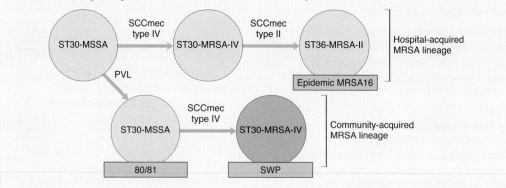

several very important questions that need to be answered. The link between virulence and specific genotypes is yet to be fully proven or disproven. Will CA-MRSA infections continue to increase as this species evolves to replace MSSA strains in the community? How do we transfer the wealth of genome and microarray data into meaningful solutions to the MRSA problem? Molecular epidemiology provides a powerful tool in our battle against this highly versatile pathogen.

Further reading

Chambers HF. The changing epidemiology of *Staphylococcus aureus*? *Emerg Infect Dis* 2001; **7**: 178–82.

Crisostomo MI, Westh H, Tomasz A *et al*. The evolution of methicillin resistance in *Staphylococcus aureus*: similarity of genetic backgrounds in historically early methicillin-susceptible and -resistant isolates and contemporary epidemic clones. *Proc Natl Acad Sci USA* 2001; **98**: 9865–70.

de Sousa MA *et al*. Intercontinental spread of a multidrug-resistant methicillin-resistant *Staphylococcus aureus* clone. *J Clin Microbiol* 1998; **36**: 2590–6.

Diep BA, Gill SR, Chang RF *et al*. Complete genome sequence of USA300, an epidemic clone of community-acquired methicillin-resistant *Staphylococcus aureus*. *Lancet* 2006; **367**: 731–9.

Ito T *et al*. Structural comparison of three types of staphylococcal cassette chromosome *mec* integrated in the chromosome in methicillin-resistant *Staphylococcus aureus*. *Antimicrob Agents Chemother* 2001; **45**: 1323–36.

Jevons MP. Celbenin-resistant staphylococci. *BMJ* 1961; **1**: 124–5.

Kravitz GR, Dries DJ, Peterson ML, Schlievert PM. Purpura fulminans due to *Staphylococcus aureus*. *Clin Infect Dis* 2005; **40**: 941–7.

Kreiswirth B, Kornblum J, Arbeit RD *et al*. Evidence for a clonal origin of methicillin resistance in *Staphylococcus aureus*. *Science* 1993; **259**: 227–30.

Miller L, Pedreau-Remington F, Rieg G *et al*. Necrotizing fasciitis caused by community-associated methicillin-resistant *Staphylococcus aureus* in Los Angeles. *N Engl J Med* 2005; **352**: 1445–-53.

Okuma K, Iwakawa K, Turnidge JD *et al*. Dissemination of new methicillin-resistant *Staphylococcus aureus* clones in the community. *J Clin Microbiol* 2002; **40**: 4289–94.

Robinson DA, Enright MC. Evolutionary models of the emergence of methicillin-resistant *Staphylococcus aureus*. *Antimicrob Agents Chemother* 2003; **47**: 3926–34.

Robinson DA, Kearns AM, Holmes A *et al*. Re-emergence of early pandemic *Staphylococcus aureus* as a community-acquired methicillin-resistant clone. *Lancet* 2005; **365**: 1256–8.

4. Epidemiology of MRSA

Jaana Vuopio-Varkila

Variation in MRSA rates
Geographic variation
MRSA situation in specific countries
MRSA carriage
Surveillance
MRSA and outbreaks

Within 2 years of the introduction of methicillin for clinical use, the first methicillin resistant *Staphylococcus aureus* was detected in England in 1961. Since then, the emergence and spread of MRSA has been documented on every continent.[1-3]

MRSA is currently the most commonly identified antibiotic-resistant pathogen in hospitals in many parts of the world, including Europe, the Americas, North Africa and the Middle and Far East.

Variation in MRSA rates

Variation in MRSA proportions exists at international and at national levels. Only a few countries are currently able to report low incidence figures for MRSA; even then, considerable variation in MRSA rates exists between hospitals within a country.[1,4,5] In Europe, in general, there is a north–south gradient, MRSA strains being relatively rare in Scandinavia and far more frequent in Southern Europe or the UK.

Many factors affect the MRSA rates (Table 4.1). In order to compare rates, the surveillance

Table 4.1
Factors that affect MRSA rates

- Baseline MRSA incidence
- Outbreaks
- Surveillance methods and their coverage
- MRSA notification systems
- Legal issues
  - Statutory versus voluntary reporting
  - Possible penalties
- Active search for MRSA patients and carriers
- MRSA sampling and screening practices
- Laboratory diagnostic techniques used for MRSA identification

methods and case identification criteria should be as identical as possible. As shown in a recent study from the US, depending on how the definition of community-acquired MRSA is formulated, the case numbers may alter significantly.[6]

Besides surveillance methods, the infrastructure of healthcare system, patient characteristics and treatment practices affect the epidemiology of MRSA. In addition, infection control resources (human and financial) and practices create differences between facilities. We have more peer-reviewed evidence on epidemiology and prevention of MRSA in acute care hospital setting than in long-term facilities, community setting or family clusters.[7-9] Table 4.2 lists factors that affect MRSA spread in hospital setting.

Table 4.2
Factors linked to spread of MRSA in hospitals

- Patient transfers within and between hospitals
- Poor communication between units
- Ignorance of recognition of risk situations or MRSA risk groups
- Increasing number of very ill patients seen in hospital
- Increasing complexity of healthcare and medical intervention
- Increasing workload and shortage of skilled staff
- Poor compliance with hand hygiene
- Difficulties in isolating patients with MRSA
- Unnecessary antibiotic usage
- New epidemic MRSA strains

MRSA trends tend to change with time.[1,4,10-12] The host and the microbe as well as the epidemiological setting are a constant target for fluctuation. Thus, typical characteristics of MRSA epidemiology may differ even within an individual healthcare facility at different times. During recent years, certain common shifts have, however, been observed:

- MRSA is no longer only linked to healthcare setting
- MRSA has become prevalent in the out-patient setting and in long-term facilities
- non-endemic countries witness rising MRSA case numbers
- MRSA strains causing infections are changing (from multiresistant to non-multiresistant)
- new risk groups for MRSA are being identified.

Geographic variation

The SENTRY programme[13] reports MRSA rates from various regions (Table 4.3). In general, the rates tend to be lower in those countries that have strict infection control policies and higher in those with more liberal or missing policies.

Similarly, the EARSS project (<http://www.rivm.nl/earss/>[5]) has followed MRSA bacteraemia rates since 1999 within the European region. The overall prevalence of MRSA bacteraemia increased between 1999 and 2004 from 16% to 24%. An increasing trend was observed in many countries, including countries with low endemicity. In 2004, the proportion of MRSA bloodstream infections was smallest in The Netherlands and the Scandinavian countries

(0–3%) and high, for example, in the UK (44%), Ireland (41%), Greece (44%) and Italy (40%).

For many less industrialised and non-industrialised countries, information on MRSA rates is limited or based on constrained case numbers. Co-incidental evidence suggests that MRSA rates may be prominent in these regions.

MRSA situation in specific countries

United States of America

The prevalence of MRSA has increased progressively since the early 1980s especially amongst hospitalised patients. MRSA has been one of the targets for the National Nosocomial Infections Surveillance (NNIS) system since its beginning. By 2004, MRSA accounted for over 60% of *S. aureus* isolations in intensive care patients.[1] Besides being a significant problem in US hospitals, MRSA is reported increasingly from the out-patient setting and from individuals without previously recognised MRSA risk factors.[11,14,15] The rapidly emerging community-acquired MRSA (CA-MRSA) has caused major concern and has even required clinicians to alter their approach to the empirical treatment of skin and soft tissue infections. Thus far, CA-MRSA has been linked to:

- children and young adults
- individuals from low socio-economic status
- day-care attendees
- prisoners
- competitive sports participants
- Native Americans
- military recruits
- men who have sex with men.

Table 4.3
Incidence of MRSA in different parts of the world (SENTRY project, 1997–1999)

Region	MRSA (%)	Low range (%)	High range (%)
Europe	1.8–54.4%	Switzerland (1.8) The Netherlands (2.0)	Italy (50.5) Portugal (54.4)
Western hemisphere	5.7–45.3%	Canada (5.7)	Chile (45.3), Argentina (42.7), USA (34.2)
Western Pacific	23.6–73.8%	Australia (23.6)	Hong Kong (73.8), Japan (71.6)

The typical CA-MRSA strains differ from hospital strains by antimicrobial resistance profile and genomic characteristics.[16] In 1992–2003, the resistance rates for several non-β-lactam antibiotics decreased also among certain hospital MRSA strains.[10]

Low numbers of vancomycin-intermediate (VISA) and vancomycin-resistant (VRSA) MRSA strains have been reported from the US since 1997.[17] There is no indication that these strains are more prone to spread than other MRSA strains. Development of a VISA or VRSA strain is linked to preceding long-term vancomycin therapy, or simultaneous VRE carriage.[18,19]

United Kingdom

MRSA is common in the UK.[1,20] A shift in the figures happened in the 1990s, from 2% in 1990 to over 40% by the turn of the century.[7] The surveillance of MRSA in the UK, a mandatory scheme run by the Department of Health, measures the number of bacteraemia cases reported by Acute NHS Trusts.[7]

The reasons for the rise in MRSA infections in the UK, as in many countries, are multifactorial. The increasing rate of children amongst the MRSA bacteraemia cases causes concern.[21,22] There is speculation that new strains that emerged in the 1990s (especially UK-EMRSA-15 and-16) may be more transmissible and virulent (i.e. more likely to cause infections) than some of their predecessors.[23,24]

The majority of MRSA cases are reported from healthcare settings; there is a lack of comprehensive data on the prevalence of CA-MRSA in England and Wales [25]. Based on current estimates, the numbers of CA-MRSA still seem to be low in the UK.[26] Information on MRSA prevalence in long-term facilities is scarce, but some centres report rather high rates.[27,28]

The Netherlands and Scandinavian countries

A common feature for all those countries that report low MRSA incidence rates is adherence to stringent MRSA control measures.[1] The tradition of active MRSA prevention measures ('search

and destroy') is well-established and in many instances endorsed by legislation. Patient records of each MRSA case are labelled accordingly, and MRSA alerts are often added to electronic patient records. The MRSA figures usually include both clinical MRSA cases and individuals who are asymptomatic MRSA carriers (such as contacts of cases). In Finland, for example, during 2001–2003, around half of the MRSA-positive patient specimens were taken on a clinical basis, and the remainder for screening after exposure to MRSA.

In spite of control efforts, increasing MRSA rates have recently been observed, especially amongst the elderly. MRSA-related problems are reported from both the out-patient setting and long-term facilities.[29–32] In Finland, the rise began after the turn of the century (Fig. 4.1). The underlying reasons were several: (i) a few healthcare facility-related MRSA outbreaks; (ii) an increasing number of MRSA cases amongst the elderly, especially in long-term facilities; and (iii) a shortage of economic and human resources. In response to the problem, the MRSA prevention guidelines were updated to cover long-term facilities and the Finnish government launched a notable fund for the health districts. As a positive sign, the MRSA figures decreased in 2005.

> Low-endemic rates reflect aggressive MRSA prevention measures.

MRSA carriage

Colonisation with MRSA results in long-term carriage. A MRSA carrier has an increased risk of developing an infection caused by MRSA.[33] The risk for MRSA transmission depends on individual predisposing risk and behavioural factors. In a high-risk setting (such as ICUs), the estimated rate of transmission can be as high as 1 to 3 and the number of secondary cases (i.e. the reproductive number) high.[34–37] Cross-transmission (patient-to-patient via transiently colonised healthcare workers) is the main means of transmission.

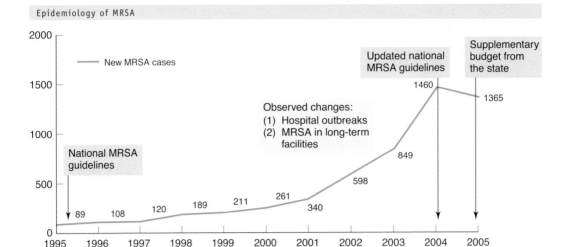

Figure 4.1
Increasing MRSA cases in Finland (1995–2005). Source: National Public Health Institute, Finland.

In the community setting, MRSA carriers represent both discharged patients and healthy individuals without conventional risk factors. Several large studies on carriage of MRSA among healthy individuals (both children and adults) have been conducted. The MRSA incidence rates are generally low (less than 1%) even in areas with high nosocomial MRSA rates.[38–43] MRSA carriage has been reported to be slightly higher in individuals over 65 years of age.[38,39] In family clusters and child day-care settings, MRSA carriage rates may turn out to be high (at least 10–15%) amongst close contacts of MRSA-positive individuals.[44–46] The scarce data on MRSA carriage rates from non-industrialised countries indicate that the problem may be significant.

Many experts recommend performance of hospital-entry MRSA screening especially for high-risk patients (based on risk-adjusted indicators).[7,47] A recent study estimated that up to 49% of MRSA carriers would have been missed without screening on admission.[48]

> The chance of becoming a MRSA carrier depends on exposure, individual predisposing risk factors and behavioural matters.

Surveillance

A functional MRSA surveillance programme: (i) provides relevant information on the extent of MRSA spread; (ii) identifies priorities for infection control and the need for adjustments; and (iii) guides antimicrobial drug policy and intervention programmes. Detection of outbreaks is strengthened by systematic surveillance. Each healthcare facility needs to plan their own MRSA surveillance scheme on the basis of local needs and resources.[7,8] An efficient MRSA surveillance scheme could consist of:

1. Collect and analyse data in a consistent way, to agreed definitions.
2. Follow results from microbiological investigations; (i) search for changes in strain profiles; (ii) observe for putative clusters; and (iii) use molecular typing as an additional epidemiological tool when indicated.
3. Feed back MRSA information to healthcare staff and management committees regularly as an integral part of the infection control programme.
4. Integrate MRSA surveillance as an element of the clinical governance process.

> The key steps in surveillance process are:
>
> - Systematic collection of data
> - Analysis
> - Interpretation
> - Dissemination for action

MRSA and outbreaks

Recognition of an outbreak may happen by chance or as a result of active MRSA surveillance. The route of transmission is sometimes impossible to track (the index case/source of infection remains unidentifiable) but, occasionally, is quite evident (a patient transfer in a low endemicity setting).[49]

MRSA outbreaks are easier to handle and control, if the number of cases is low and the spread is limited. Evidence comes particularly from facilities with low baseline MRSA figures and where an active 'search and destroy' MRSA prevention policy is conducted.[49–52] Several studies have shown that outbreak investigation and consecutive control measures are cost effective, at least in situations when MRSA has not reached endemic rates.[53,54]

> Early recognition of an outbreak leads to better outcome.

References

1. Boyce JM, Cookson B, Christiansen K et al. Methicillin-resistant Staphylococcus aureus. Lancet Infect Dis 2005; 5: 653–63.

2. Zinn CS, Westh H, Rosdahl VT, Sarisa Study Group. An international multicenter study on antimicrobial resistance and typing of hospital Staphylococcus aureus isolates from 21 laboratories in 19 countries or states. Microb Drug Resist 2004; 10: 160–8.

3. Kesah C, Ben Redjeb S, Odugbemi TO et al. Prevalence of methicillin-resistant Staphylococcus aureus in eight African hospitals and Malta. Clin Microbiol Infect 2003; 9: 153–6.

4. Chambers HF. The changing epidemiology of Staphylococcus aureus? Emerg Infect Dis 2001; 7: 178–82.

5. Tiemersma EW, Bronzwaer SL, Lyytikäinen O et al; European Antimicrobial Resistance Surveillance System

Participants. Methicillin-resistant Staphylococcus aureus in Europe, 1999–2002. Emerg Infect Dis 2004; 10: 1627–34.

6. Folden DV, Machayya JA, Sahmoun AE et al. Estimating the proportion of community-associated methicillin-resistant Staphylococcus aureus: two definitions used in the USA yield dramatically different estimates. J Hosp Infect 2005; 60: 329–32.

7. Coia JE, Duckworth GJ, Edwards DI et al; Joint Working Party of the British Society of Antimicrobial Chemotherapy; Hospital Infection Society; Infection Control Nurses Association. Guidelines for the control and prevention of meticillin-resistant Staphylococcus aureus (MRSA) in healthcare facilities. J Hosp Infect 2006; 63: S1–44.

8. Gould IM. The clinical significance of methicillin-resistant Staphylococcus aureus. J Hosp Infect 2005; 61: 277–82.

9. Loveday HP, Pellowe CM, Jones SR, Pratt RJ. A systematic review of the evidence for interventions for the prevention and control of methicillin-resistant Staphylococcus aureus (1996–2004): report to the Joint MRSA Working Party (Subgroup A). J Hosp Infect 2006; 63: S45–70.

10. Klevens RM, Edwards JR, Tenover FC, McDonald LC, Horan T, Gaynes R; National Nosocomial Infections Surveillance System. Changes in the epidemiology of methicillin-resistant Staphylococcus aureus in intensive care units in US hospitals, 1992–2003. Clin Infect Dis 2006; 42: 389–91.

11. Zetola N, Francis JS, Nuermberger EL, Bishai WR. Community-acquired methicillin-resistant Staphylococcus aureus: an emerging threat. Lancet Infect Dis 2005; 5: 275–86.

12. Chambers HF. Community-associated MRSA – resistance and virulence converge. N Engl J Med 2005; 352: 1485–7.

13. Fluit AC, Wielders CL, Verhoef J, Schmitz FJ. Epidemiology and susceptibility of 3,051 Staphylococcus aureus isolates from 25 university hospitals participating in the European SENTRY study. J Clin Microbiol 2001; 39: 3727–32.

14. Shopsin B, Mathema B, Martinez J et al. Prevalence of methicillin-resistant and methicillin-susceptible Staphylococcus aureus in the community. J Infect Dis 2000; 182: 359–62.

15. Weber JT. Community-associated methicillin-resistant Staphylococcus aureus. Clin Infect Dis 2005; 41: S269–72.

16. Vandenesch F, Naimi T, Enright MC et al. Community-acquired methicillin-resistant Staphylococcus aureus carrying Panton-Valentine leukocidin genes: worldwide emergence. Emerg Infect Dis 2003; 9: 978–84.

17. Cosgrove SE, Carroll KC, Perl TM. Staphylococcus aureus with reduced susceptibility to vancomycin. Clin Infect Dis 2004; 39: 539–45.

18. Centers for Disease Control and Prevention (CDC). Vancomycin-resistant Staphylococcus aureus – New York, 2004. MMWR Morb Mortal Wkly Rep 2004; 53: 322–3.

19. Whitener CJ, Park SY, Browne FA et al. Vancomycin-resistant Staphylococcus aureus in the absence of vancomycin exposure. Clin Infect Dis 2004; **38**: 1049–55.

20. Griffiths C, Lamagni TL, Crowcroft NS, Duckworth G, Rooney C. Trends in MRSA in England and Wales: analysis of morbidity and mortality data for 1993–2002. Health Stat Q 2004; **Spring**: 15–22.

21. Khairulddin N, Bishop L, Lamagni TL, Sharland M, Duckworth G. Emergence of methicillin resistant Staphylococcus aureus (MRSA) bacteraemia among children in England and Wales, 1990–2001. Arch Dis Child 2004; **89**: 378–9.

22. Adedeji A, Gray JW. MRSA at an English children's hospital from 1998 to 2003. Arch Dis Child 2005; **90**: 720–3.

23. Robinson DA, Kearns AM, Holmes A et al. Re-emergence of early pandemic Staphylococcus aureus as a community-acquired methicillin-resistant clone. Lancet 2005; **365**: 1256–8.

24. Johnson AP, Aucken HM, Cavendish S et al; UK EARSS participants. Dominance of EMRSA-15 and -16 among MRSA causing nosocomial bacteraemia in the UK: analysis of isolates from the European Antimicrobial Resistance Surveillance System (EARSS). J Antimicrob Chemother 2001; **48**: 143–4.

25. Health Protection Agency. Community MRSA in England and Wales: definition through strain characterization. Commun Dis Rep Wkly [serial online] 15 March 2005; **15**: News. Available at:<http://www.hpa.org.uk/cdr/archives/2005/cdr1105.pdf>.

26. Holmes A, Ganner M, McGuane S, Pitt TL, Cookson BD, Kearns AM. Staphylococcus aureus isolates carrying Panton-Valentine leukocidin genes in England and Wales: frequency, characterization, and association with clinical disease. J Clin Microbiol 2005; **43**: 2384–90.

27. Maudsley J, Stone SP, Kibbler CC et al. The community prevalence of methicillin-resistant Staphylococcus aureus (MRSA) in older people living in their own homes: implications for treatment, screening and surveillance in the UK. J Hosp Infect 2004; **57**: 258–62.

28. Morgan M, Evans-Williams D, Salmon R, Hosein I, Looker DN, Howard A. The population impact of MRSA in a country: the national survey of MRSA in Wales, 1997. J Hosp Infect 2000; **44**: 227–39.

29. Kerttula A-M, Lyytikäinen O, Salmenlinna S, Vuopio-Varkila J. Changing epidemiology of methicillin-resistant Staphylococcus aureus in Finland. J Hosp Infect 2004; **58**: 109–14.

30. Stenhem M, Ortqvist A, Ringberg H et al; Swedish Study Group on MRSA Epidemiology. Epidemiology of methicillin-resistant Staphylococcus aureus (MRSA) in Sweden 2000–2003, increasing incidence and regional differences. BMC Infect Dis 2006; **6**: 30.

31. Wertheim HF, Vos MC, Boelens HA et al. Low prevalence of methicillin-resistant Staphylococcus aureus (MRSA) at hospital admission in The Netherlands: the value of search and destroy and restrictive antibiotic use. J Hosp Infect 2004; **56**: 321–5.

32. Faria NA, Oliveira DC, Westh H et al. Epidemiology of emerging methicillin-resistant Staphylococcus aureus (MRSA) in Denmark: a nationwide study in a country with low prevalence of MRSA infection. J Clin Microbiol 2005; **43**: 1836–42.

33. von Eiff C, Becker K, Macha K et al. Nasal carriage as a source of Staphylococcus aureus bacteremia. N Engl J Med 2001; **344**: 11–6.

34. Grundmann H, Hori S, Winter B, Tami A, Austin DJ. Risk factors for the transmission of methicillin-resistant Staphylococcus aureus in an adult intensive care unit: fitting a model to the data. J Infect Dis 2002; **185**: 481–8.

35. Marshall C, Harrington G, Wolfe R, Fairley CK, Wesselingh S, Spelman D. Acquisition of methicillin-resistant Staphylococcus aureus in a large intensive care unit. Infect Control Hosp Epidemiol 2003; **24**: 322–6.

36. Regev-Yochay G, Rubinstein E, Barzilai A et al. Methicillin-resistant Staphylococcus aureus in neonatal intensive care unit. Emerg Infect Dis 2005; **11**: 453–6.

37. Bootsma MC, Diekmann O, Bonten MJ. Controlling methicillin-resistant Staphylococcus aureus: quantifying the effects of interventions and rapid diagnostic testing. Proc Natl Acad Sci USA 2006; **103**: 5620–5.

38. Kuehnert MJ, Kruszon-Moran D, Hill HA et al. Prevalence of Staphylococcus aureus nasal colonization in the United States, 2001–2002. J Infect Dis 2006; **193**: 172–9.

39. Graham 3rd PL, Lin SX, Larson EL. A U.S. population-based survey of Staphylococcus aureus colonization. Ann Intern Med 2006; **144**: 318–25.

40. Sa-Leao R, Sanches IS, Couto I, Alves CR, de Lencastre H. Low prevalence of methicillin-resistant strains among Staphylococcus aureus colonizing young and healthy members of the community in Portugal. Microb Drug Resist 2001; **7**: 237–45.

41. Zanelli G, Sansoni A, Zanchi A et al. Staphylococcus aureus nasal carriage in the community: a survey from central Italy. Epidemiol Infect 2002; **129**: 417–20.

42. Hisata K, Kuwahara-Arai K, Yamanoto M et al. Dissemination of methicillin-resistant staphylococci among healthy Japanese children. J Clin Microbiol 2005; **43**: 3364–72.

43. Huang YC, Su LH, Chen CJ, Lin TY. Nasal carriage of methicillin-resistant Staphylococcus aureus in school children without identifiable risk factors in northern Taiwan. Pediatr Infect Dis J 2005; **24**: 276–8.

44. Shahin R, Johnson IL, Jamieson F, McGeer A, Tolkin J, Ford-Jones EL. Methicillin-resistant Staphylococcus aureus carriage in a child care center following a case of disease. Toronto Child Care Center Study Group. Arch Pediatr Adolesc Med 1999; **153**: 864–8.

45. Eveillard M, Martin Y, Hidri N, Boussougant Y, Joly-Guillou ML. Carriage of methicillin-resistant *Staphylococcus aureus* among hospital employees: prevalence, duration, and transmission to households. *Infect Control Hosp Epidemiol* 2004; **25**: 114–20.

46. Jensen JU, Jensen ET, Larsen AR *et al.* Control of a methicillin-resistant *Staphylococcus aureus* (MRSA) outbreak in a day-care institution. *J Hosp Infect* 2006; **63**: 84–92.

47. Eveillard M, Leroy C, Teissiere F *et al.* Impact of selective screening in the emergency department on methicillin-resistant *Staphylococcus aureus* control programmes. *J Hosp Infect* 2006; **63**: 380–4.

48. Harbarth S, Sax H, Fankhauser-Rodriguez C, Schrenzel J, Agostinho A, Pittet D. Evaluating the probability of previously unknown carriage of MRSA at hospital admission. *Am J Med* 2006; **119**: 275.e15–23.

49. Duckworth GJ, Lothian JL, Williams JD. Methicillin-resistant *Staphylococcus aureus*: report of an outbreak in a London teaching hospital. *J Hosp Infect* 1988; **11**: 1–15.

50. Kotilainen P, Routamaa M, Peltonen R *et al.* Eradication of methicillin-resistant *Staphylococcus aureus* from a health center ward and associated nursing home. *Arch Intern Med* 2001; **161**: 859–63.

51. Kotilainen P, Routamaa M, Peltonen R *et al.* Elimination of epidemic methicillin-resistant *Staphylococcus aureus* from a university hospital and district institutions, Finland. *Emerg Infect Dis* 2003; **9**: 169–75.

52. Pastila S, Sammalkorpi KT, Vuopio-Varkila J, Kontiainen S, Ristola MA. Control of methicillin-resistant *Staphylococcus aureus* outbreak involving several hospitals. *J Hosp Infect.* 2004; **58**: 180–6.

53. Vriens M, Blok H, Fluit A, Troelstra A, Van Der Werken C, Verhoef J. Costs associated with a strict policy to eradicate methicillin-resistant *Staphylococcus aureus* in a Dutch University Medical Center: a 10-year survey. *Eur J Clin Microbiol Infect Dis* 2002; **21**: 782–6.

54. Bjorholt I, Haglind E. Cost-savings achieved by eradication of epidemic methicillin-resistant *Staphylococcus aureus* (EMRSA)-16 from a large teaching hospital. *Eur J Clin Microbiol Infect Dis* 2004; **23**: 688–95.

5. MRSA at home and on the farm

Andreas Voss, Margreet C Vos

Defining non-healthcare acquired MRSA

Epidemiology

Prevention of CA-MRSA and CO-MRSA

MRSA in animals

Since the first report on methicillin-resistant *Staphylococcus aureus* (MRSA) in 1961,[1] MRSA has steadily increased in prevalence and become a global problem. It soon became clear that outbreaks occurred in hospitals as early as 1968. While the prevalence of MRSA may still significantly differ between different regions and countries, MRSA has become endemic around the world and may cause up to 60% of all *S. aureus* infections.[2,3] For more than 40 years, MRSA infections were more or less exclusively seen among hospitalised patients with multiple risk factors.[4] The first CA-MRSA mainly included non-acute care hospital-associated MRSA and included large numbers of cases from skilled nursing facilities and dialysis centres. More recently, however, MRSA infections have been described in patients without established risk factors for MRSA.[5-7]

> In a population-based study, Kuehnert et al.[8] recently found that 0.8% harboured MRSA which would translate to 2.3 million persons in the US.

One of the first reports, showing the dramatic consequences of this emerging disease in populations not expected to acquire this disease, was the description of four children in Minnesota and North Dakota, who died from severe MRSA infections.[9] The emergence of community-acquired MRSA (CA-MRSA) requires reconsideration of current epidemiological definitions and risk groups. It is remarkable that, at opposite sides of the world, the problem of CA-MRSA arose more or less at the same time and at the same magnitude – the US, Canada and Australia.[10-13] The driving forces and epidemiology of this phenomenon need well-designed, community-based studies which include adequate risk factors.

Other newly discovered niches of MRSA are household pets and cattle. This chapter describes both the epidemiological changes of CA-MRSA, the presence of MRSA in animals and the possible link between the two.

Defining non-healthcare acquired MRSA

Until recently, there was no need to describe or define further MRSA strains with regard to their origin, since carriage, onset of infections and outbreaks were mainly limited to hospitalised patients, or those recently treated in healthcare centres. While the increasing prevalence in hospitalised patients can obviously lead to a spill-over into the community (thereby appearing in close contact with formerly hospitalised patients), an increasing number of reports of MRSA in patients that lack any classical risk-factor for MRSA carriage indicate a change in the epidemiology. Most of the infections concerned were soft tissue and skin infections. With this increase in reports, it became clear that we urgently need clear definitions to be able to define exactly the magnitude of the problem and identify risk factors. In the literature, different terms and definitions are used. This has led to at least three terms; community-acquired, community-associated (CA) or community onset (CO)-MRSA[14] and it is often unclear whether authors have made a distinction between community-acquired/associated and community-onset MRSA.

Some definitions of CA-MRSA are solely based on the place and time of their first detection.

According to this 'epidemiological definition', all MRSA isolates found in out-of-hospital patients or those admitted to a hospital for less than 48–72 hours, are community-acquired. Furthermore, the first detection can be a colonising strain, or the strain causing clinical infection. Since colonisation may occur within the first hours after admission and/or may persist for a long time after hospitalisation,[15] the place of first detection is a poor attribute to define CA-MRSA, and may obviously differ from the place the first contact with MRSA occurred.[16] Consequently, the problem of CA-MRSA is overestimated using an epidemiological definition.[14,17,18] Other definitions were based on the absence of recent hospitalisation, or the lack of typical nosocomial risk-factors for MRSA colonisation.[19-21] However, these determinants too were not able to define the problem of CA-MRSA and may actually lead to an underestimation.[14,22]

Others have used molecular characteristics to describe CA-MRSA. However, molecular attributes, such as the presence of SCCmec type IV cannot be used as part of the definition of CA-MRSA, as strains harbouring these molecular properties can be found and transmitted in either a healthcare centre (HCC) or outside in the community. Furthermore, although many strains found in the community harbour the Panton-Valentin leukocidin (PVL) genes and, therefore, assumed to be more virulent, the possession of the gene should not be part of the definition of CA-MRSA.[23,24] Next to the small, rather mobile SCCmec type IV and PVL genes, susceptibility to most antibiotics other than β-lactam have been associated with CA-MRSA strains. For these molecular and susceptibility characteristics, the same holds true as for the presence of SCCmec type IV; their presence is more common in strains spreading in the community, but cannot serve as (part of) a definition, but at most can be used as an alert or indication of probable CA-MRSA.

For the most part, authors refer to community-acquired in either new, unexpected outbreaks of infections by MRSA in populations not linked to HCCs by MRSA strains not formerly known to have caused nosocomial outbreaks (i.e. newly emerging strains or based on the timing of isolation. Community-onset refers mostly to the place where transmission of MRSA occurred (i.e. the community).

Before identifying a single infection or an outbreak to be of community origin, and not HCC associated, source finding and molecular typing methods are needed.

> The best definition of CA-MRSA is probably the combination of epidemiological features, source finding and molecular typing.

When using this combined epidemiological and molecular definition, it is found that most CA-MRSA: (i) are susceptible to most antibiotics other than β-lactams; (ii) have genotypes that do not match HA-MRSA strains; (iii) are SCCmec type IV; and (iv) harbour PVL genes. The patients involved show no hospital-associated risk factors.[25,26]

Ultimately, the MRSA problem will rise in time as 'real' CA-MRSA may spread to healthcare workers[27] and/or hospitalised patients,[28] thereby leading to colonisation or infection of truly hospitalised patients.

To achieve uniformity, we recommend the following definitions.

MRSA

mecA-Positive S. aureus strains with altered penicillin-binding protein (PBP2a), irrespective of phenotypic susceptibility to β-lactam or the genotypic and/or phenotypic susceptibility to other antibiotics.

Staphylococcal cassette chromosome mec (SCCmec)

The mobile element integrated in the S. aureus chromosome, harbouring the mecA gene. Currently five types of SSCmec have been identified,[29,30] which differ in size and composition. The origin of SSC*mec* in *S aureus* probably lies in coagulase-negative staphylococci.[29] SSC*mec* has entered *S. aureus* on a limited number of occasions and can be found in several clonal lineages world-wide.[28]

Hospital-acquired MRSA (HA-MRSA)

Carriage of, or infection with, MRSA strains, acquired in a HCC (*i.e.* a hospital setting, a long-term care facility or an out-patient clinic). Detection is mostly after 48 hours of admission; detection within 48 hours of admission should carefully be explored on possible transmission within the first 48 hours, or during a (out-patient) visit or prior admission to a HCC. HA-MRSA can easily be introduced into the community, and transmitted to others.[17] For precise discrimination between HA-MRSA, CA-MRSA and CO-MRSA, the moment in time of transmission and the source should be identified by contact tracing and molecular typing.

Community-acquired MRSA (CA-MRSA)

This definition should be a combination of the following three characteristics.

1. Carriage of, or infections with, MRSA first detected in a patient outside healthcare institutions, or within the first 48 hours of admission; AND

2. No epidemiological relation, such as having been treated in a HCC in the previous year, or being a close contact of a carrier-patient in the previous year or carrier-HCW (preferable excluded by contact search); AND

3. The following molecular characteristics are present: SCC*mec* type IV or V, and phylogenetically unrelated to previously known HA-MRSA lineages.

Given this definition, CA-MRSA are formerly methicillin sensitive *S. aureus* (MSSA) strains which have acquired the SSC*mec* and transmit from one to the other in communities prone to selection (antibiotic use) and/or close contact (*e.g.* sports, jails, child-care facilities). The lineages of HA-MRSA are distinct from those defined as CA-MRSA.[23] The introduction of SSC*mec* into sensitive clones is most likely a relatively infrequent event.[31] Carriers of CA-MRSA can introduce, if undetected and/or if no adequate preventive measures are taken, these strains into the HCCs. The evolution of such strains will be by acquiring resistance to other antibiotic agents,[32] the reason why antibiotic resistance profiles are not part of our definition of CA-MRSA. In future, it is to be expected that successful CA-MRSA clones will become the next generation of successful (multiresistant) HA-clones, as occurred with the paediatric clone in Portugal.[31]

Given the discussion with regard to the definition of CA-MRSA and the possibility of HA-MRSA and CA-MRSA spreading in the community or in healthcare settings, respectively, the authors believe that using this 3-part definition of CA-MRSA is probably the best to describe and determine the recent change in the epidemiology and clinical presentations of MRSA infections.

Community-onset MRSA (CO-MRSA)

Genetically unrelated or related with known HA-MRSA or CA-MRSA strains, but found in patients lacking classical MRSA risk-factors and no contact with healthcare institutions, including long-term facilities and out-patient clinics in the previous year. CO refers to the place where transmission occurred; this is, by definition, the community and can involve a typical HA-MRSA or CA-MRSA strain. Thus, 'by definition', CO-MRSA includes some HA-MRSA present in the community, next to all truly CA-MRSA. CO-MRSA is not limited to certain MRSA lineages, SSC*mec*-types or other characteristics, but solely describes the place of transmission.

Epidemiology

The main change with regard to MRSA around the world is the fact that MRSA carriage and infection are no longer limited to healthcare institutions.

MRSA carriage and infection are increasingly reported in healthy individuals who have little or no contact with healthcare settings and. therefore, lack classical healthcare-associated risk-factors for MRSA.[9,14,28,33-35] Although CA-MRSA infections are frequently mild skin and soft-tissue infections, severe life-threatening and lethal cases of necrotising pneumonia, fasciitis, and bloodstream infections, have been reported.[36,37]

> Transmission of CA-MRSA, leading to community outbreaks, so far has primarily been reported in specific populations, such as jail inmates, aboriginals, soldiers, athletes, sports-clubs, men who have sex with men, and children in childcare.[38-45]

One of the first reports of the spread of MRSA in the community is that of Saravolatz et al.[46] describing, over a 19- month period, an outbreak of 165 patients with MRSA infections in the Detroit area. They noticed, in March 1980, 3% of community-acquired S. aureus infections being methicillin resistant; this percentage gradually increased to 38% in 1981. In their study, they defined nosocomial infections as occurring with onset 72 hours after a patient had entered the hospital, or being related to an intervention occurring during the first 72 hours of hospitalisation. All infections by MRSA not identified as nosocomial were considered as community-acquired. They found that parenteral drug abusers comprised 61% of all patients with MRSA infections. Only 12% of abusers with MRSA were hospitalised during the year before they developed MRSA infection; in contrast, 65% of all non-abuser MRSA patients had been hospitalised. Using their definition of CA-MRSA by exclusion, they probably overestimated the proportion of CA-MRSA. However, hospitalised drug abusers with no infection had a nasal carriage rate of MRSA of 11%, whereas HCWs had a carriage rate of 0.7%. Previous antibiotic use had a significant association with CA-MRSA and, in an earlier study, they found that excessive use of antibiotics among this particular population

appear to play a major role in acquiring MRSA. It was clear that transmission of MRSA occurred in the closed community of drug abusers, probably brought into that community from the hospital. The authors concluded that control measures in the hospital will have little effect on the community reservoir and MRSA may replace MSSA in their area.

So far, it is uncertain whether specific risk-factors for CA-MRSA colonisation or infection exist. While some authors describe younger age as a risk factor,[23] any difference in age between MRSA and CA-MRSA patients may be explained by different settings (i.e. the selective population of the hospitalised patient). Still, the impact on the treatment of staphylococcal infections in children is huge, since in some areas as much as 75% of all community-associated staphylococcal infections are caused by MRSA.[47] Creech et al.[48] reported a MRSA colonisation rate of 9.2% among healthy US children. Furthermore, in their region, the MRSA prevalence rate among healthy children increased by more than 10-fold between 2001 and 2004.[48]

Prior use of antibiotics has been reported as a possible risk factor,[42,49] but other investigators could not confirm this finding.[50] Naimi et al.[51] compared the epidemiological and molecular differences of 1100 MRSA patients and the infecting MRSA strains. They used an epidemiological definition of no medical history within 1 year of the MRSA culture date. SSI infections were more common in the CA-group, and CA-patients were significantly younger.

Now, some data are available on the true prevalence of MRSA in the population. In countries with a very low prevalence of nosocomial strains, like The Netherlands, repeated prevalence studies on diverse populations hardly indicated any MRSA carriers,[52,53] although small outbreaks of transmission of CA-MRSA in The Netherlands have occurred.[54] This could be a reflection of the active 'search and destroy' policy, which has been in use for many years.[55-58] However, countries with high rates of HA-MRSA and reports of outbreaks of CA-MRSA still have low prevalence rates when measured in the healthy population. Recently, data from the US show that in the healthy community this rate was 0.84%.[59,60] Furthermore, in a meta-analysis, it was shown that among community members without healthcare contacts, the pooled MRSA colonisation rate was 0.2%.[14] In Portugal, the prevalence of MRSA nasal carriage was found to be 0.7%, measured in young and healthy individuals from the community;[61] in Switzerland, CA-MRSA upon admission to the hospital has been reported to be 0.1%.[50]

Data on the prevalence in communities of different countries are still rather sparse, despite the large number publications on the topic from around the world. Obviously, the prevalence per region or country differs, as it does for HA-MRSA. In each prevalence study performed, the problem of using different definitions arises, which makes the studies difficult to compare. Determining prevalence rates of CA-MRSA in hospitalised patients with infections, instead of members of the community, may lead to an overestimate of its occurrence.[14] In a meta-analysis, Saldago *et al.*[14] found prevalence rates of more than 30% in 32 studies of hospitalised patients with CA-MRSA, whereas the prevalence was only 0.2% in healthy individuals without healthcare contacts.

The chances are that the epidemiology of CA-MRSA will be more difficult to describe in the future, since truly community-acquired strains may spread to healthcare workers and/or be transmitted between patients,[27,28] actually leading to a replacement of hospital-acquired MRSA in some hospitals.[16] In any case, the occurrence of CA-MRSA and CO-MRSA may have a major impact on the overall prevalence and control of MRSA. Some authors fear that the history of penicillin-resistant *S. aureus* may repeat itself.[33] Once these strains reached a high prevalence in hospitals (as MRSA has done today in most countries), transmission into the community began, leading to replacement of penicillin-susceptible strains.

Thus the occurrence of CA-MRSA and CO-MRSA may just be a repeat of history, only that today penicillin-resistant, methicillin-susceptible *S. aureus* (MSSA) strains are replaced by MRSA.

At the same time, a completely reverse process may occur, namely the spread of CA-MRSA within hospitals[16,62] as well as the occurrence of CA-MRSA and CO-MRSA entirely unrelated to healthcare.[27]

Possibly, the latest occurrences of CA-MRSA in countries with a low prevalence of MRSA may help to get better insight into the onset and epidemiology of CA-MRSA. In The Netherlands and Scandinavia, the prevalence of MRSA in clinical isolates of *S. aureus* has been < 1% over the past decade[52] and is still one of the lowest in Europe if not the world.[55] This low prevalence is best explained by the 'search and destroy' policy applied by these countries, which demands isolation and screening of all patients at risk of MRSA carriage before admission to a hospital.[57] In the past, 'at-risk' patients mainly consisted of patients who had been admitted to and/or treated in hospitals foreign to the above mentioned countries. When the occurrence of non-healthcare related MRSA strains in the community increases, this poses a risk to the 'search and destroy' policy. In this case, the policy need to be adapted to new 'risk-groups' over time.

Prevention of CA-MRSA and CO-MRSA

Prevention of CA-MRSA

There are no published data on the prevention of new emerging strains. However, logically and bearing in mind the definition above, prevention of CA-MRSA starts with prevention of picking up SSC*mec* genes by successful MSSA clones from methicillin-resistant coagulase-negative staphylococci (MRSE). Unfortunately, it is not known what the driving force to this process is. However, antibiotic use selects for MRSE in the community, and thus increases the burden of *mecA*; it sounds logical that prudent use of antibiotics lowers the chance of the emergence of new MRSA strains. Obviously, we need more studies on the origins and risk factors of these new strains. Once CA-MRSA emerges, prevention measures should be installed to resolve the outbreak (see below).

> Most CA-MRSA infections present with skin and soft tissue infections in the community.

An important preventive measure is to educate people how to limit transmission from infections, including basic hygienic measures in wound care. Information should be given to the patient, the caregivers and close contacts regarding precautions in wound care and hand hygiene in the home. Learning theory suggests that compliance with contact precautions for CA-MRSA may be greater than for traditional HA-MRSA infection or colonisation. This is because the patient with CA-MRSA usually has a physical manifestation of their disease. However, this applies to the index patient and close contacts who contract a 'visible' infection, but not for those who become a carrier. Unfortunately, carriers act as a source of transmission to others as well. Further, it is to be expected that patients, after being cured from their infection, remain nasal carriers, and thus remain infectious.

Prevention of CO-MRSA

> A prerequisite for the prevention of CO-MRSA is knowledge of infected, and thus infectious, people.

Patients with HA-MRSA discharged from HCCs should be identified and followed up. Recently, in The Netherlands, a national policy was developed to prevent transmission of MRSA in the community to risk groups. Risk groups are those with underlying diseases making them prone to staphylococcal disease, or being a patient with regular visits to HCCs, or being a healthcare worker, or a close contact to one of these (Fig. 5.1). These 'at risk' persons are

strongly advised to undergo eradication therapy and, until successfully performed, be treated in accordance with Dutch infection control measures in HCCs, as described in the national guideline of the 'search and destroy' strategy (<www.wip.nl>, <www.infectieziekten.info>). Eradication therapy should be initiated as soon as possible. Eradication therapy should not be performed if the patient has wounds or catheters in place, as eradication is less successful in these cases. Successful eradication therapy is the cornerstone of prevention of transmission in the community as people cannot be excluded from having social contacts. The most successful eradication strategy, however, includes detection of all carriers within a closed community (e.g. a family or household) and treatment of all carriers at the same time. If this procedure is not followed, the chance of re-infection from a close contact is possible. In our experience, transmission of HA-MRSA within a family occurs in 50% of cases. Agreement should be achieved between public health, primary care and hospital personnel to indicate responsibilities for contact tracing, and for the choice, indication and administration of eradication therapy; decisions should be made on who takes care of the follow-up cultures after therapy.

MRSA in animals

Until recently, it was assumed that methicillin resistance was absent from staphylococci isolated from animals. In a prevalence study, van Duijkeren et al. reported a low prevalence of MRSA among staphylococci isolated from animals. Among 10 mecA positive staphylococci, only two were MRSA, both cultured from dogs. Overall, there are few reports on infections of animals with MRSA. In Korea, Japan, Belgium, the UK, The Netherlands, and the US, infections with MRSA have been reported in horses, dogs and cattle. Given the fact that food animals and household pets have different risk factors for the occurrence (e.g. antibiotic use) and transmission (e.g. petting) of MRSA, these kind of animals are discussed separately.

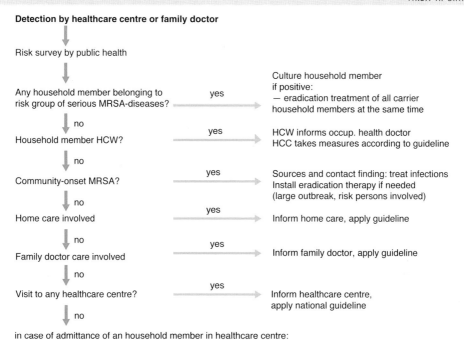

Detection by healthcare centre or family doctor

Risk survey by public health

Any household member belonging to risk group of serious MRSA-diseases? — yes → Culture household member if positive:
— eradication treatment of all carrier household members at the same time

no ↓

Household member HCW? — yes → HCW informs occup. health doctor
HCC takes measures according to guideline

no ↓

Community-onset MRSA? — yes → Sources and contact finding: treat infections
Install eradication therapy if needed
(large outbreak, risk persons involved)

no ↓

Home care involved — yes → Inform home care, apply guideline

no ↓

Family doctor care involved — yes → Inform family doctor, apply guideline

no ↓

Visit to any healthcare centre? — yes → Inform healthcare centre, apply national guideline

no ↓

in case of admittance of an household member in healthcare centre: warn the centre

Figure 5.1
Actions to be performed by public health authority after the finding of MRSA, either HA, CO or CA. Based on Dutch national guideline (<www.infectieziekten.info>).

Small animals/household pets

In household animals, MRSA infections have been uncommon, but are increasing, possibly due to the increasing prevalence of human MRSA in the community.

Especially with household pets, such as cats and dogs, the transmission of MRSA in general seems to be from human to the animal. While such animals may initially be colonised by their owners, they may become a source of re-infection, as described by van Duijkeren *et al.* when a nurse (and family) carried an epidemic HA-MRSA after repeated unsuccessful decolonisation treatment and only became MRSA-free after the family dog was included in the decolonisation treatment. Transmission between owner and pet dog have also been reported in the US.

Loeffler *et al.* looked at the relatedness between human and animal isolates among veterinary staff and animals in a small animal hospital in the UK. MRSA was found in 18% of the staff (*n* = 14), 9% of the animals (*n* = 4 dogs) and 10% of the environmental samples (*n* = 3). More than 80% of the MRSA isolates were indistinguishable, or closely related to, one of the UK epidemic MRSA strains (EMRSA-15), possibly indicating a common source. However, the mode by which EMRSA-15 was introduced into the hospital remained unclear. In this local, epidemic situation, the prevalence of MRSA among the veterinary staff was significantly higher than for the UK health community.

Food animals

In a Korean study of major food animals, the prevalence of MRSA among *S. aureus* isolates was 3.6%. The majority (13 of 15) of the MRSA isolates were found in milk specimens of dairy cattle. No MRSA were found among isolates from beef cattle and pigs. Nine of the 12 dairy cattle had an infection (mastitis).

In France, Aubry-Damon et al. determined the association between contact with pigs and isolation of antimicrobial-resistant micro-organisms comparing healthy pig farmers to non-farmers, each matched for sex, age, and county of residence. The prevalence of nasal or pharyngeal isolation of S. aureus was nearly 2 times higher in pig farmers. Since the prevalence of S. aureus nasal carriage in non-farmers was similar to that reported earlier, the authors concluded that the higher isolation rate in pig farmers was due to their work environment. Their hypothesis was further supported by the nearly 10-times increased resistance to macrolides, which is the fourth most common class of antimicrobial agents used in food production in France. Five pig farmers (4.4%), but no non-farmers, carried MRSA.

In The Netherlands recently, the link between pig-farming and MRSA in humans was further established. The occurrence of unexpected cases of MRSA in the hospital setting was linked to patients that had direct contact with pigs or were part of the immediate family of a pig-farmer. MRSA cases, related to the pig-strain, included colonised patients and patients with soft tissue and skin infections.

> In one region with 9 out of 10 pigs infected, all family members of the farmer and all co-workers on the farm were MRSA positive.

In one region, 23% of the regional pig-farmers were MRSA carriers, thereby exceeding the prevalence of MRSA in the general population by more than 700-fold. Following this initial observation, a representative portion of Dutch pigs were screened and shown to harbour MRSA (average ~40%, range 0–100% for different batches). While obviously further research is needed into other food animals, most

importantly we need to know the risk of those humans who are occupationally exposed to pigs (and possible other food animals). This is of utmost importance in order to prevent failure of the Dutch 'search and destroy' policy for MRSA. Among Dutch veterinarians in contact with pigs and cattle, the carriage of MRSA was shown to be close to 5%, equivalent to the rate of carriage among patients returning from foreign hospitals who presently are isolated and screened on admission to Dutch hospitals, according to the 'search and destroy' policy.

In addition to the finding of MRSA in colonised, living animals and from infectious sites, MRSA has been isolated from raw, retail chicken meat in Japan. The risk of transfer of MRSA from raw meat to consumers remains to be assessed. Furthermore, the question remains whether the chicken meat were intrinsically colonised, or if the meat was contaminated during processing.

> Before drawing final conclusions, more research on food animals and their handlers is needed. In particular, the influence of antibiotic-use needs to be established. The MRSA strain in Dutch pigs, for example, is in nearly all cases resistant to tetracycline, an antibiotic frequently used in pig-farming.

References

1. Jevons MP. Celbenin-resistant Staphylococci. *BMJ* 1961; **1**: 124–6.
2. Tiemersma EW, Bronzwaer SLAM, Lyytikäinen O *et al.*; and European Antimicrobial Resistance Surveillance System Participants. Methicillin-resistant *Staphylococcus aureus* in Europe, 1999–2002. *Emerg Infect Dis* 2004; **10**: 1627–33.
3. National Nosocomial Infections Surveillance System. National Nosocomial Infections Surveillance (NNIS) System Report, data summary from January 1992 through June 2004, issued October 2004. *Am J Infect Control* 2004; **32**: 470–85.
4. Thompson RL, Cabezudo I, Wenzel RP. Epidemiology of nosocomial infections caused by methicillin-resistant *Staphylococcus aureus*. *Ann Intern Med* 1982; **97**: 309–17.
5. Coombs GW, Pearson JC, O'Brien FG *et al.* Methicillin-resistant *Staphylococcus aureus* clones, Western Australia. *Emerg Infect Dis* 2006; **12**: 241–7.

6. Carleton HA, Diep BA, Charlebois ED, Sensabaugh GF, Perdreau-Remington F. Community-adapted methicillin-resistant *Staphylococcus aureus* (MRSA): population dynamics of an expanding community reservoir of MRSA. *J Infect Dis* 2004; **190**: 1730–8.

7. Kluytmans-Vandenbergh MF, Kluytmans JA. Community-acquired methicillin-resistant *Staphylococcus aureus*: current perspectives. *Clin Microbiol Infect* 2006; **12 (Suppl 1)**: 9–15.

8. Kuehnert MJ, Kruszon-Moran D, Hill HA *et al*. Prevalence of *Staphylococcus aureus* nasal colonization in the United States, 2001–2002. *J Infect Dis* 2006; **193**: 172–9.

9. Centers for Disease Control and Prevention. Four pediatric deaths from community-acquired methicillin-resistant *Staphylococcus aureus* – Minnesota and North Dakota, 1997–1999. JAMA 1999; **282**: 1123–5.

10. Fridkin SK, Hageman JC, Morrison M *et al*. Methicillin resistant *Staphylococcus aureus* disease in three communities. *N Engl J Med* 2005; **352**: 1436–44.

11. Stevenson KB, Searle K, Stoddard G *et al*. Methicillin-resistant *Staphylococcus aureus* and vancomycin-resistant Enterococci in rural communities, western United States. *Emerg Infect Dis* 2005; **11**: 895–903.

12. Mulvey MR, MacDougall L, Cholin B *et al* Community-associated methicillin-resistant *Staphylococcus aureus*, Canada. *Emerg Infect Dis* 2005; **6**: 844–50.

13. Coombs GW, Nimmo GR, Bell JM *et al*. Genetic diversity among community methicillin-resistant *Staphylococcus aureus* strains causing outpatient infections in Australia. *J Clin Microbiol* 2004; **42**: 4735–43.

14. Salgado CD, Farr BM, Calfee DP. Community-acquired methicillin-resistant *Staphylococcus aureus*: a meta-analysis of prevalence and risk factors. *Clin Infect Dis* 2003; **36**: 131–9.

15. Sanford MD, Widmer AF, Bale MJ, Jones RN, Wenzel RP. Efficient detection and long-term persistence of the carriage of methicillin-resistant *Staphylococcus aureus*. *Clin Infect Dis* 1994; **19**: 1123–8.

16. Turnidge JD, Bell JM. Methicillin-resistant *Staphylococcus aureus* evolution in Australia over 35 years. *Microb Drug Resist* 2000; **6**: 223–9.

17. Charlebois ED, Perdreau-Remington F, Kreiswirth B *et al*. Origins of community strains of methicillin-resistant *Staphylococcus aureus*. *Clin Infect Dis* 2004; **39**: 47–54.

18. Folden DV, Macahyya JA, Sahmoun AE *et al*. Estimating the proportion of community-associated methicillin-resistant *Staphylococcus aureus*: two definitions used in the USA yield dramatically different estimates. *J Hosp Infect* 2005; **60**: 329–32.

19. Liao CH, Chen SY, Chang SC *et al*. Characteristics of community-acquired and health care-associated *Staphylococcus aureus* bacteremia in patients treated at the emergency department of a teaching hospital. *Diagn Microbiol Infect Dis* 2005; **53**: 85–92.

20. Okuma K, Iwakawa K, Turnidge JD *et al*. Dissemination of new methicillin-resistant *Staphylococcus aureus* clones in the community. *J Clin Microbiol* 2002; **40**: 4289–94.

21. Chambers HF. Community-associated MRSA – resistance and virulence converge. *N Engl J Med* 2005; **352**: 1485–7.

22. Naimi TS, LeDell KH, Como-Sabetti K *et al*. Comparison of community- and health care-associated methicillin-resistant *Staphylococcus aureus* infection. *JAMA* 2003; **290**: 2976–84.

23. Vandenesch F, Naimi T, Enright MC *et al*. Community-acquired methicillin-resistant *Staphylococcus aureus* carrying Panton-Valentine leukocidin genes: worldwide emergence. *Emerg Infect Dis* 2003; **9**: 978–84.

24. Robinson DA, Enright MC. Evolutionary models of the emergence of methicillin-resistant *Staphylococcus aureus*. *Antimicrob Agents Chemother* 2003; **47**: 3926–34.

25. Enright MC, Robinson DA, Randle G *et al*. The evolutionary history of methicillin-resistant *Staphylococcus aureus* (MRSA). *Proc Natl Acad Sci USA* 2002; **99**: 7687–92.

26. Voss A, Loeffen F, Bakker J, Wulf M, Klaassen C. Methicillin-resistant *Staphylococcus aureus* in pig farming. *Emerg Infect Dis* 2005; **11**: 1965–6.

27. Ochoa TJ, Mohr J, Wanger A, Murphy JR, Heresi GP. Community-associated methicillin-resistant *Staphylococcus aureus* in pediatric patients. *Emerg Infect Dis* 2005; **11**: 966–8.

28. Ito T, Ma XX, TakeuchiF, Okuma K, Yuzawa H, Hiramatsu K. Novel type V staphylococcal cassette chromosome *mec* driven by a novel cassette chromosome recombinase, *ccrC*. *Antimicrob Agents Chemother* 2004; **48**: 2637–51.

29. Wu SW, DE Lencastre H, Tomasz A. Recruitment of the *mecA* gene homologue of *Staphylococcus sciuri* into a resistance determinant and expression of the resistant phenotype in *Staphylococcus aureus*. *J Bacteriol* 2001; **183**: 2417–24.

30. Aires de Sousa M, Conceicao T, Simas C *et al*. Comparison of genetic backgrounds of methicillin-resistant and - susceptible *Staphylococcus aureus* isolates from Portuguese hospitals and the community. *J Clin Microbiol* 2005; **43**: 5150–7.

31. Deresinski S. Methicillin-resistant *Staphylococcus aureus*: an evolutionary, epidemiologic, and therapeutic odyssey. *Clin Infect Dis* 2005; **40**: 562–73.

32. Chambers HF. The changing epidemiology of *Staphylococcus aureus*? *Emerg Infect Dis* 2001; **7**: 178–82.

33. King MD, Humphrey BJ, Wang YF *et al*. Emergence of community-acquired methicillin-resistant *Staphylococcus aureus* USA 300 clone as the predominant cause of skin and soft-tissue infections. *Ann Intern Med* 2006; **144**: 309–17.

34. Gorak EJ, Yamada SM, Brown JD. Community-acquired methicillin-resistant *Staphylococcus aureus* in hospitalized adults and children without known risk factors. *Clin Infect Dis* 1999; **29**: 797–800.

35. Durand G, Bes M, Meugnier H et al. Detection of new methicillin-resistant Staphylococcus aureus clones containing the toxic shock syndrome toxin 1 gene responsible for hospital- and community-acquired infections in France. Clin Microbiol 2006; 44: 847–53.

36. Maltezou HC, Giamarellou H. Community-acquired methicillin-resistant Staphylococcus aureus infections. Int J Antimicrob Agents 2006; 27: 87–96.

37. Centers for Disease Control and Prevention. Outbreaks of community-associated methicillin-resistant Staphylococcus aureus skin infections – Los Angeles County, California, 2002–2003. MMWR Morb Mortal Wkly Rep 2003; 52: 88.

38. Maguire GP, Arthur AD, Boustead PJ, Dwyer B, Currie BJ. Clinical experience and outcome of community-acquired and nosocomial methicillin-resistant Staphylococcus aureus in a northern Australian hospital. J Hosp Infect 1998; 38: 273–81.

39. Centers for Disease Control and Prevention. Community-associated methicillin-resistant Staphylococcus aureus infections in pacific islanders – Hawaii, 2001–2003. MMWR Morb Mortal Wkly Rep 2004; 53: 767–70.

40. Zinderman CE, Conner B, Malakooti MA, LaMar JE, Armstrong A, Bohnker BK. Community-acquired methicillin-resistant Staphylococcus aureus among military recruits. Emerg Infect Dis 2004; 10: 941–4.

41. Ellis MW, Hospenthal DR, Dooley DP, Gray PJ, Murray CK. Natural history of community-acquired methicillin-resistant Staphylococcus aureus colonization and infection in soldiers. Clin Infect Dis 2004; 39: 971–9.

42. Kazakova SV, Hageman JC, Matava M et al. A clone of methicillin-resistant Staphylococcus aureus among professional football players. N Engl J Med 2005; 352: 468–75.

43. Nguyen DM, Mascola L, Brancoft E. Recurring of methicillin-resistant Staphylococcus aureus infections in a football team. Emerg Infect Dis 2005; 11: 526–532.

44. Adcock PM, Pastor P, Medley F, Patterson JE, Murphy TV. Methicillin-resistant Staphylococcus aureus in two child care centers. J Infect Dis 1998; 178: 577–80.

45. Saravolatz LD, Donald J, Pohlod MS et al. Community-acquired methicillin resistant Staphylococcus aureus infections: a new source for nosocomial outbreaks. Ann Intern Med 1982; 97: 325–9.

46. Kaplan S, Hulten KG, Gonzales BE et al. Three-year surveillance of community-acquired Staphylococcus aureus infections in children. Clin Infect Dis 2005; 40: 1785–91.

47. Creech CB, Talbot TR, Schaffner W. Community-associated methicillin-resistant Staphylococcus aureus: the way to the wound is through the nose. J Infect Dis 2006; 193: 169–71.

48. Baggett HC, Hennessy TW, Leman R et al. An outbreak of community-onset methicillin-resistant Staphylococcus aureus skin infections in southwestern Alaska. Infect Control Hosp Epidemiol 2003; 24; 397–402.

49. Harbarth S, François P, Schrenzel J et al. Community-associated methicillin-resistant Staphylococcus aureus, Switzerland. Emerg Infect Dis 2005; 11: 962–5.

50. Naimi TS, LeDell KH, Boxrud DJ et al. Epidemiology and clonality of community-acquired methicillin-resistant Staphylococcus aureus in Minnesota, 1996–1998. Clin Infect Dis 2001; 33: 990–6.

51. Wertheim HF, Vos MC, Boelens HA et al. Low prevalence of methicillin-resistant Staphylococcus aureus (MRSA) at hospital admission in The Netherlands: the value of search and destroy and restrictive antibiotic use. J Hosp Infect 2004; 56: 321–5.

52. Melles DC, Gorkink RF, Boelens HA et al. Natural population dynamics and expansion of pathogenic clones of Staphylococcus aureus. J Clin Invest 2004; 114: 1732–40.

53. Wannet WJ, Spalburg E, Heck ME et al. Emergence of virulent methicillin-resistant Staphylococcus aureus strains carrying Panton-Valentine leukocidin genes in The Netherlands. J Clin Microbiol 2005; 43: 3341–5.

54. Voss A, Milatovic D, Wallrauch-Schwarz C, Rosdahl VT, Braveny I. Methicillin-resistant Staphylococcus aureus in Europe. Eur J Med Microbiol Infect Dis 1994; 13: 50–5.

55. Vos MC, Verbrugh HA. MRSA: we can overcome, but who will lead the battle? Infect Control Hosp Epidemiol 2005; 26: 117–20.

56. Verhoef J, Beaujean D, Blok H et al. A Dutch approach to methicillin-resistant Staphylococcus aureus. Eur J Clin Microbiol Infect Dis 1999; 18: 461–6.

57. EARSS Annual Report 2004. ISBN-number 90-6960-131-1 (<www.earss.rivm.nl>).

58. Kuehnert MJ, Kruszon-Moran D, Hill HA et al. Prevalence of Staphylococcus aureus nasal colonization in the United States, 2001–2002. J Infect Dis 2006; 193: 172–9.

59. Graham 3rd PL, Lin SX, Larson EL. A U.S. population-based survey of Staphylococcus aureus colonization. Ann Intern Med 2006; 144: 318–25.

60. Sa-Leao R, Sanches IS, Couto I, Alves CR, de Lencastre H. Low prevalence of methicillin-resistant strains among Staphylococcus aureus colonizing young and healthy members of the community in Portugal. Microb Drug Resist 2001; 7: 237–45.

61. Seybold U, Kourbatova EV, Johnson JG et al. Emergence of community-associated methicillin-resistant Staphylococcus aureus USA300 genotype as a major cause of health care-associated blood stream infections. Clin Infect Dis 2006; 42: 647–56.

Further reading for MRSA in animals

Aubry-Damon H, Grenet K, Sall-Ndiaye P et al. Antimicrobial resistance in commensal flora of pig farmers. Emerg Infect Dis 2004; 10: 873–9.

Devrieze LA, Hommez J. Epidemiology of methicillin-resistant Staphylococcus aureus in dairy herds. Res Vet Sci 1975; 19: 23–7.

Gortel K, Campbell KL, Kakoma I, Whittem T, Schaeffer DJ, Weisiger RM. Methicillin resistance among staphylococci isolated from dogs. *Am J Vet Res* 1999; **60**: 1526–30.

Hartmann FA, Trostle SS, Klohnen AA. Isolation of methicillin-resistant *Staphylococcus aureus* from a postoperative wound infection in a horse. *J Am Vet Med Assoc* 1997; **211**: 590–2.

Kitai S, Shimizu A, Kawano J, Sato E, Nakano C, Uji T, Kitagawa H. Characterization of methicillin-resistant *Staphylococcus aureus* isolated from retail raw chicken meat in Japan. *J Vet Med Sci* 2005; **67**: 107–10.

Loeffler A, Boag AK, Sung J *et al.* Prevalence of methicillin-resistant *Staphylococcus aureus* among staff and pets in a small animal referral hospital in the UK. *J Antimicrob Chemother* 2005; **56**: 692–7.

Manian FA. Asymptomatic nasal carriage of mupirocin-resistant, methicillin resistant *Staphylococcus aureus* (MRSA) in a pet dog associated with MRSA infection in household contacts. *Clin Infect Dis* 2003; **36**: E26–8.

Moulin G. Surveillance of antimicrobial consumption: activities in France (Agence Nationale du Médicament Vétérinaire). In: 2nd International Conference of the Office International des Epizoosties, 2001; Paris; 2001.

Pak SI, Han HR, Shimizu A., Characterization of methicillin-resistant *Staphylococcus aureus* isolated from dogs in Korea. *J Vet Med Sci* 1999; **61**: 1013–8.

Seguin JC, Walker RD, Caron JP *et al.* Methicillin-resistant *Staphylococcus aureus* outbreak in a veterinary teaching hospital: potential human-to-animal transmission. *J Clin Microbiol* 1999; **37**, 1459–63.

Shimizu A, Kawano J, Yamamoto C, Kakutani O, Anzai T, Kamada M. 1997. Genetic analysis of equine methicillin-resistant *Staphylococcus aureus* by pulsed-field gel electrophoresis. *J Vet Med Sci* 1997; **59**, 935–7.

Tomlin J, Pead MJ, Lloyd DH *et al.* Methicillin-resistant *Staphylococcus aureus* infections in 11 dogs. *Vet Rec* 1999; **144**: 60–4.

Van Duijkeren E, Wolfhagen MJ, Box AT, Heck ME, Wannet WJ, Fluit AC. Human-to-dog transmission of methicillin-resistant *Staphylococcus aureus*. *Emerg Infect Dis* 2004; **10**: 2235–7.

van Duijkeren E, Box AT, Heck ME, Wannet WJ, Fluit AC. Methicillin-resistant staphylococci isolated from animals. *Vet Microbiol* 2004; **103**: 91–7.

Weese JS. Methicillin-resistant *Staphylococcus aureus*: an emerging pathogen in small animals. *J Am Animal Hosp Assoc* 2005; **41**: 150–7.

6. MRSA – advances in laboratory detection, identification and antibiotic susceptibility testing

Donald Morrison

Rapid MRSA laboratory reporting
Molecular basis of methicillin resistance
Laboratory detection and confirmation of MRSA
Conclusions

MRSA constitutes a major public health threat and presents both a therapeutic and an infection control challenge in the hospital setting and, more recently, in the community. In combating this threat, the clinical microbiology laboratory plays a pivotal role in the detection, identification and antibiotic-susceptibility testing of MRSA. Timely antibiotic susceptibility results inform clinicians regarding treatment options and rapid MRSA diagnosis provides essential data for preventing transmission. With the advent in recent years of new, especially molecular, testing methods, issues relating to the most appropriate laboratory tests for MRSA diagnosis are currently under debate. Although molecular methods promise to revolutionise infectious disease diagnosis, their implementation into the laboratory faces considerable hurdles including expensive equipment and reagents, technical expertise and a major work-flow shift

to facilitate their introduction. These new assays, however, present the laboratory with tests which could have a significant impact on the control of MRSA.

> Molecular methods promise to revolutionise infectious disease diagnosis; However, their implementation faces considerable hurdles.

Rapid MRSA laboratory reporting

MRSA diagnosis in the laboratory may, at present, take up to 5 days and few doubt that rapid reporting would significantly improve outcomes both for individual infected patients and rates of hospital-acquired infections. In fact, several studies have shown that infected patients obtain more rapid adjustment of therapy leading to a decrease in mortality, reduction in the use of vancomycin, shorter hospital length of stay and the inevitable decrease in costs for the hospital. One study reported that 39% of blood-culture positive patients were on ineffective empirical therapy. Another found that 25% of patients received a change of therapy following rapid reporting. Five patients with MSSA were switched from vancomycin to oxacillin, one with methicillin-resistant coagulase-negative staphylococci (MR-CoNS) was started on vancomycin, and one with MR-CoNS was switched from a cephalosporin plus vancomycin to vancomycin alone regimen. Surprisingly, two other patients confirmed with MSSA were continued on vancomycin therapy! Rapid reporting is also critical for effective infection control and will contribute significantly in limiting the spread of MRSA in the hospital environment.

> A mathematical model has shown that rapid diagnostic testing for MRSA can reduce isolation needs by > 90% in low-endemic settings and by 20% in high-endemic settings.

A Swiss study compared conventional 4-day detection of MRSA with a rapid 23-hour molecular method and found that a strategy linking the rapid screening test to pre-emptive isolation and cohorting of MRSA patients substantially reduced MRSA cross-infections in the medical ICU. In addition, the added effort required for contact precautions and isolation measures can be more adequately targeted saving resources and stress on patients who are subjected to these measures unnecessarily. In an article titled *Let MRSA-positive patients live a normal life*, it has been argued that isolation may have potentially negative consequences. Surprisingly, one group found that isolated patients were less likely than other patients to be examined by physicians during rounds.

Several obstacles need to be overcome for rapid reporting to be introduced in the clinical microbiology laboratory, not least of which is the cost element. Rapid tests are more expensive than conventional ones; for molecular techniques, the cost implications are significant. At costs of up to £15 for a rapid molecular test and with some laboratories screening over 100 MRSA swabs per day, it is clear that this would be a major financial burden for the laboratory.

> If costs are considered on a hospital wide, rather than individual department, basis, then the introduction of rapid tests would give an overall cost benefit to the hospital.

A study on a related hospital pathogen found that real-time PCR detection of vancomycin-resistant enterococci reduced patients 'length of stay' by 2 days and saved the hospital an estimated $205,000 per year. The cost and workload involved in MRSA screening can be reduced considerably if specimens from different sites are pooled but this may result in reduced test sensitivity. Screening a single site, such as the nose, would also reduce cost and workload but again with a likely reduction in sensitivity.

Molecular basis of methicillin resistance

All *Staphylococcus aureus* strains produce four major cell wall enzymes (penicillin binding protein 1, PBP 2, PBP 3, and PBP 4) which are involved in the cross-linking of peptidoglycan, an integral component of the bacterial cell wall. The β-lactam antibiotics bind with high affinity to these PBPs, inactivate their cross-linkage function, inhibit cell wall formation and kill the bacteria. By definition, all MRSA contain a 'foreign', non-*S. aureus*, gene designated *mecA* which encodes for a PBP with low affinity for β-lactam antibiotics. This PBP, designated PBP2a or PBP2′, can function in the presence of high concentrations of β-lactam antibiotics, enabling cell wall cross-linkage and survival of cells. The *mecA* gene is part of a much larger genetic element termed staphylococcal cassette chromosome *mec* (SCC*mec*) which is thought to have been acquired from a MR-CoNS. However, the data to support this are not, as yet, conclusive.

Heterogeneous resistance

> A major problem in the laboratory diagnosis of MRSA is the nature of the phenotypic expression of methicillin resistance.

Four resistance expression classes have been described: Class 4, or homogeneous resistant strains, where every cell in a culture are highly resistant (minimum inhibition concentration [MIC] $\geq$ 800 mg/l) and Classes 1, 2, and 3 which have a heterogeneous form of resistance where a culture consists of subpopulations of cells with differing levels of resistance expression. MIC for Classes 1, 2 and 3 range from 1.5–3 mg/l, 6–12 mg/l and 50–200 mg/l, respectively. In heterogeneous strains, the majority of cells are susceptible to low concentrations of β-lactam antibiotics (less than the breakpoint) and only a small proportion of cells (1 in 10^6) can grow at high concentrations. However, under antibiotic pressure, even Class 1 strains can give rise to cultures of highly resistant cells; from a clinical perspective, every MRSA, irrespective of its expression Class, can potentially cause treatment failure *in vivo*. Although homogeneously resistant isolates are identified accurately in the laboratory, many clinical isolates express resistance heterogeneously and this continues to be a challenge to the clinical microbiology laboratory.

The basis for heterogeneous resistance in MRSA is multifactorial. Mutations in the *mecA* promoter region or *mecI* polymorphisms may result in heterogeneous resistance. In addition, many MRSA have partial deletion of the regulatory genes and PBP2a production in these strains is constitutive. However, if the strain carries an inducible β-lactamase plasmid, the β-lactamase regulatory genes are able to co-regulate PBP2a production. In MRSA with intact and fully functional *mec* regulatory genes, the production of PBP2a is strongly repressed and they will appear susceptibility by conventional testing. These are termed 'preMRSA' and are thought to be rare. However, as these isolates possess the *mecA* gene, they should be treated as 'MRSA' in terms of therapy and infection control decisions. In addition, several other mechanisms, including the *fem* (factors essential for methicillin resistance) or *aux* (auxillary) genes, the global regulators (*agr* and *sar*) and other chromosomal genes have been associated with heterogeneous resistance. Many of these mechanism are only partially understood.

Borderline resistance

Heterogeneous methicillin resistance can result in false-negative results and another phenomenon, often designated 'borderline' resistance, can lead to false positive results. BORSA (borderline oxacillin resistance *S. aureus*) have low level methicillin resistance with MIC at, or just above, the susceptibility breakpoint but, importantly, are *mecA* negative. There is some confusion in terminology as BORSA has also been used to designate heterogeneous resistance MRSA. Borderline resistance in *mecA*-negative strains has been attributed to either penicillinase hyper-production or modification of the PBPs normally carried by *S. aureus*. These latter strains have also been termed MODSA (moderately resistant *S. aureus*). Significantly, it does not appear that the low level of resistance

expressed by *mecA*-negative borderline strains leads to treatment failure.

Laboratory detection and confirmation of MRSA

It is a little surprising given the threat and publicity surrounding MRSA over the last decade that only recently have we seen progress in the rapid laboratory diagnosis of MRSA. Two developments, the introduction of cefoxitin as a surrogate marker for methicillin resistance and the unravelling of the SCC*mec* element following MRSA genome sequencing, have been particularly significant.

There are now three choices available to the clinical microbiology laboratory for the laboratory diagnosis of MRSA: (i) conventional reporting (2–3 day method); (ii) next-day reporting; and, most significantly, (iii) same-day reporting.

Conventional MRSA laboratory reporting (2–3 day method)
Solid media culture (1–2 days)

Although clinical samples may be plated directly onto a non-selective blood agar media, it is common to use a selective media for MRSA detection in the laboratory. These media contain: (i) an indicator to distinguish *S. aureus*; (ii) an inhibitory substance to suppress other organisms; and (iii) methicillin or oxacillin to select methicillin-resistant isolates. One of the distinguishing features of *S. aureus* is its ability to grow in high-salt concentrations and this is the commonest inhibitory agent used in selective media with levels as high as 7% NaCl being used. However, care is required as some *S. aureus*, notably strains of EMRSA-16, the second commonest MRSA clone in the UK, may be inhibited at such high concentrations. Fermentation of mannitol, detected by pH change, is the commonest indicator and Mannitol Salt Agar (MSA) with or without methicillin or oxacillin, or variations of this medium, such as ORSAB (oxacillin resistance screening agar base), have been used extensively to screen for MRSA.

Other screening media such as Baird Parker and Columbia Blood agar with various selective agents have also been used. Although MRSA may be detected on MSA/ORSAB at 24 hours, the sensitivity is low (49%) and further incubation, for up to 48 hours, is required to increase sensitivity (69%). The specificity of MSA/ORSAB media is around 92%. Baird Parker Ciprofloxacin media may give sensitivities of 74% and 90% at 24 and 48 hours, respectively.

Enrichment culture (2–3 days)

Enrichment broths, which may include inhibitory and selective agents such as NaCl and methicillin/oxacillin, are used to increase sensitivity by allowing small numbers of MRSA to grow during an overnight incubation step before plating on agar media. Enrichment is suitable for screening to ensure clearance of MRSA in high-risk patients or in low prevalence areas and is the method of choice in many Dutch hospitals where the prevalence of methicillin resistance amongst S. aureus is < 1%. Enrichment, however, introduces a further time delay. Indicator-enrichment media which also include a means of detecting growth without further subculture, can reduce workloads; if the media has high negative predictive value (NPV), then negative broths can be reported immediately without further work. However, this usually requires up to 48 hours' incubation. One study took this concept a step further and looked at indicator-enrichment media in a 'bedside screening test' model. Nurses inoculated the media, incubation was on the ward and reading was performed by the nursing staff. This test had a NPV of 99% and proved to be a useful, rapid, and inexpensive tool for the early implementation of measures to prevent the spread of MRSA.

MRSA confirmation (1 day)

It is important to distinguish S. aureus from coagulase-negative staphylococci (CoNS). This is especially so as up to 80% of hospital CoNS may be methicillin resistant.

Latex agglutination tests are simple, rapid (< 5 minutes) and the most widely used method to identify S. aureus to the species level. These tests detect surface antigens of S. aureus and there are at least 6 commercial kits on the market with sensitivities of 89–100% and specificities of 91–99%. However, as with most tests, false-positive and false-negative results may be obtained. Several CoNS may give false positive results including Staphylococcus intermedius, Staphylococcus lugdunensis, Staphylococcus schleiferi, Staphylococcus saprophyticus and Staphylococcus hyicus. Interestingly, lower sensitivity is observed with MRSA than with MSSA. The tube coagulase test which detects free (extracellular) coagulase is the 'gold standard' phenotypic method and, although results can be read at 4 hours, negative tests should be re-examined at 24 hours. Rare strains are negative in this test. The DNase test is cost effective and can be used to screen large numbers of isolates easily; however, it is less specific than latex with some CoNS giving positive results. The slide coagulase test, which detects bound coagulase (clumping factor), is simple but up to 15% of S. aureus are negative. Several biochemical identification kits are available including automated systems such as the Vitek and Phoenix. These give good performance but are more expensive and time consuming than the other methods and are seldom used to identify S. aureus. A new test kit, Staphychrom II, is a 2-hour test and good sensitivity and specificity have been reported. A commercial molecular identification kit, the AccuProbe Staphylococcus aureus Culture Identification Test, is also available for species' identification of S. aureus.

It is well known that several conditions used in phenotypic in vitro laboratory tests are known to affect the expression of resistance. These include the test agent, media, incubation temperature and time, inoculum size and NaCl concentration. Methicillin is thought to be better than oxacillin as a test agent; however, it is no longer manufactured. Muller-Hinton and Columbia agar media are more reliable than Iso-Sensitest and addition of up to 5% NaCl improves detection of resistance. Both the CLSI (USA) and BSAC (UK) recommend the addition of 2% NaCl. Detection of resistance is more reliable at lower temperature such as 30°C. As some heterogeneous strains may grow slowly, incubation for up to 48 hours may improve detection; the BSAC and CLSI standardised methods require that tests using oxacillin or methicillin should be incubated for a full 24 hours rather than the 16–20 hours used for other antibiotic susceptibility tests.

> The introduction of cefoxitin for antibiotic susceptibility testing was a major advance in the laboratory detection of MRSA.

Cefoxitin has been shown conclusively to be a more reliable surrogate marker of MRSA than oxacillin. One major advantage of cefoxitin is that, unlike methicillin/oxacillin, the optimum test conditions (Iso-sentist or Muller–Hinton agar, no added NaCl, 35°C incubation temperature, 18–20 hour incubation time) are similar to what can be used in the clinical microbiology laboratory for susceptibility testing of other antibiotics. It is, however, critical that the incubation temperature must not exceed 36°C; this is important, as in some laboratories antibiotic susceptibility testing was carried out at 37°C rather than 35°C. A further advantage of cefoxitin is that 'borderline' MSSA (hyper-β-lactamase producers) are clearly distinguished as sensitive on this test. Several concentration of cefoxitin have been tested including 5 µg, 10 µg and 30 µg. The 30 µg discs are used in the US with Muller-Hinton agar but were thought to produce too large a zone with Iso-Sensitest agar in Europe. The BSAC recommend the use of a 10 µg disc and a zone breakpoint of ≥ 22 mm indicating sensitivity.

Antibiotic susceptibility testing by the disk diffusion method is easy to set up and cost effective; it is the most widely used method for confirming methicillin resistance in clinical microbiology laboratories. Agar and broth dilution methods which will give a MIC result

are also used but are more laborious. The Etest method also gives a MIC result and is as easy to set up as disk diffusions. Breakpoint methods are similar to dilution MIC methods but test only the breakpoint concentration (2 mg/l oxacillin, 4 mg/l methicillin) and a standardised form of the breakpoint method has been recommended by the CLSI: Muller-Hinton agar, 4% NaCl, 6 mg/l oxacillin, 35°C for a full 24 hour. In addition, several automated systems including Vitek, Phoenix and Microscan are available and are generally reported as reliable.

Next day MRSA laboratory reporting

Although several studies have attempted to develop methods which will give an MRSA diagnosis on the next day, these have been restricted to a few laboratories. Recent developments such as the introduction of cefoxitin and commercially available chromogenic MRSA screening media are significant advances which have the potential for allowing clinical microbiology laboratories to adopt a 'next-day' MRSA diagnosis.

Chromogenic media (18–24 hours)

Cefoxitin, a cephamcyin antibiotic which is a good inducer of methicillin resistance, has also been shown to be superior to oxacillin and methicillin as a selective agent in both agar and broth screening media. Chromogenic MRSA screening media use cefoxitin to select for MRSA, foster better growth of MRSA and, crucially, provide good sensitivity at 18–24 hours rather than at 48 hours. In the last few years, four commercially available chromogenic media have been evaluated: MRSA Select (BioRad), CHROMagar (Becton Dickinson), MRSA ID (BioMeriuex) and Chromogenic MRSA Agar (Oxoid). In early studies, these media appear to be clearly superior to MSA with sensitivity and specificity of > 95% and > 99.8%, respectively, at 24 hours. At 48 hours, these media may be less specific and at least one of them is reported to give inferior results with perineum swabs. They may not inhibit all other organisms, such as enterococci, but the inclusion of a chromogen enables differentiation of species by colour. Some of these media require to be stored and incubated in the dark as prolonged exposure to light may result in reduced coloration of colonies. Although the cost of these media are higher than traditional media, it is likely that with increased use the cost will decrease. It is claimed by some that chromogenic media can achieve isolation and presumptive identification of MRSA in a single step with no need for additional tests to confirm the presence of MRSA.

MRSA confirmation (15 minutes to 4 hours)

Until the 'single-step, direct reporting' claims for these chromogenic media are substantiated, many microbiologists will not be satisfied without undertaking confirmatory tests. There are at least four commercial non-PCR based and several in-house or commercial PCR-based assays available which will confirm MRSA status in 15 minutes to 4 hours, hence allowing 'next-day' MRSA reporting. The four non-PCR assays are easy to use, require no special equipment and can fit easily into a routine clinical microbiology laboratory work-flow. The **MRSA-Screen PBP2a latex agglutination** is a simple, rapid and cost-effective assay which detects PBP2a, the *mecA* gene product. This test developed in 1998 by a Japanese company (Denka Seiken Co) is supplied by two UK companies (as Mastalex and PBP2a Latex Agglutination) and was a very important development for rapid reporting of MRSA. It is a 10-minute slide agglutination test using latex particles sensitised with a monoclonal antibody against PBP2a and is superior to any single phenotype-based susceptibility testing method. With sensitivity and specificity of > 98 and $\geq$ 99%, respectively, it approaches the accuracy of PCR-based *mecA* detection methods. Isolates producing small amounts of PBP2a may give weak or slow reactions but testing with a larger inoculum or following induction of PBP2a by growth in the presence of methicillin/oxacillin can resolve these issues.

Growth on media containing high NaCl concentration may affect this test; however, data from one of these chromogenic media, containing 2.5% NaCl, suggest that this was not a problem. The **Velogene Rapid MRSA assay** is the nearest rival to the PBP2a latex in terms of speed with results available in 1.5 hours or an estimated 20 tests in 2 hours. Developed in 1999, this test uses a microtray format which can be read by visual inspection or spectrophotometrically but unlike PBP2a latex, directly detects the *mecA* gene. It also gives similar sensitivity (98.5%) and specificity (100%) to PBP2a latex. The **EVIGENE MRSA Detection kit**, developed in 1999, is a colorimetric gene probe hybridisation assay for the detection of the *mecA* and *nuc* genes in a microwell strip format. The inclusion of the *S. aureus* specific *nuc* gene allows the simultaneous identification of *S. aureus* and methicillin resistance in one assay. It is a highly reliable method for MRSA and especially for borderline resistant strains. The **BBL Crystal MRSA ID System** is a 4-hour assay; unlike the other non-PCR methods, it is a selective growth based method. Growth in an oxacillin broth culture is detected via a fluorescent indicator which detects the presence of dissolved oxygen. Sensitivity and specificity of 99% and 98%, respectively, have been reported; however, as this method is dependant on the phenotypic expression of resistance, it is more prone to misclassification of borderline resistance strains.

Recognising that many laboratories may not be able to adopt high-cost methods, a simple, cost-effective, colorimetric, growth-based detection has been developed using either resazurin or a nitrate reductase assay to detect MRSA in a microtitre tray format. Although preliminary results look promising, further evaluation is required. While automated systems such as the Vitek-2 and Phoenix provide species' identification within 4 hours, antibiotic susceptibility testing requires up to 7 hours and for oxacillin may require longer. In addition, automated systems may struggle to distinguish borderline resistant isolates. The 'prototype' CytAMP MRSA assay is another clinical microbiology laboratory user-friendly assay which detects a *S. aureus* specific gene and the *mecA* gene in a 3.5 hour microtray format assay using isothermal amplification.

PCR-based methods are the 'gold standard' for identification of MRSA providing rapid and unambiguous results and these have been used routinely as the standard method for identification of MRSA in reference laboratories. It is possible, although rare, that PCR *mecA* positive isolates may carry a non-functional or non-expressed *mecA* and that new strains may have functional *mecA* which lack the PCR assay primer target sequence, thus giving rise to false positive and negative results. The PCR assay can also be affected by various inhibitors and should, therefore, include an internal control. In-house, 3-hour, conventional, gel-based PCR or 1-hour, real-time PCR methods have been used successfully in conjunction with an overnight broth enrichment step to generate sensitive and specific 'next-day' results. The relatively higher costs, specialist equipment and technical expertise required for in-house PCR methods mean that few clinical microbiology laboratories can adopt these methods. One Swedish laboratory has used a real-time PCR assay for routine MRSA screening and with a 'next-day' NPV of 99.6% has saved on the labour and reagent costs usually required for further processing of these samples. The Genotype MRSA (Hain Lifescience), a commercial kit which uses PCR and DNA Strip technology (described below), can identify MRSA from pure culture in 2 hours.

Blood cultures MRSA confirmation

Rapid reporting of positive blood cultures are crucial for patient care. The PBP2a latex agglutination test has been evaluated; however, poor sensitivity was obtained when used directly on positive blood cultures. Several studies have evaluated the ability of molecular methods to detect MRSA rapidly direct from positive blood cultures with promising results – in some assays within 4 hours. At least three

commercial kits are available. The EVIGENE MRSA Detection kit has been used in conjunction with a 3-hour enrichment step and results were obtained within 7 hours. The GenoType BC Gram-positive (Hain Lifescience) based on DNA Strip technology (described below) allows the detection of 17 Gram-positive bacterial species and resistance to methicillin and vancomycin within a few hours. The hyplex BloodScreen BSP (BAG-BiologischeAnalysensystem GmbH), a microtray format assay (described below), can detect six Gram-positive bacterial species and resistance to methicillin from a positive blood culture within 5 hours.

Same-day MRSA laboratory reporting

> Same-day detection of MRSA direct from clinical samples is the optimal detection method. The development of such assays has been hampered because the *mecA* gene is highly conserved in all species of staphylococci and primers used to detect *mecA* in *S. aureus* will also detect *mecA* in CoNS.

It is important to distinguish MRSA from MR-CoNS and some of these assays use primers to detect a *S. aureus* specific gene in addition to the *mecA* gene. However, such assay will give MRSA positive results when tested on a mixed culture of an MSSA and a MR-CoNS. Importantly, up to 80% of hospital CoNS are methicillin resistance. Although the occurrence of such mixed cultures is low in blood cultures this is not the case for the non-sterile sites used in MRSA screening.

Five assays, four of which are commercially available, have been developed and are at different stages of evaluation. In these assays, four different strategies have been adopted to enable 'same-day' MRSA reporting: selective enrichment/immunomagnetic separation (BacLite Rapid MRSA); immunomagnetic separation/PCR amplification (Immunocapture-coupled PCR assay); simultaneous detection of MR-CoNS (hyplex *Staphylo*Resist); and the

SCCmec right extremity/*orfX* junction approach (GenoType MRSA Direct and IDI MRSA). The latter is both novel and promising and is based on the region where SCC*mec* integrates into the MSSA chromosome. This region comprises the right extremity region of SCC*mec*, the SCC*mec* integration site and the *orfX* gene – a gene carried by all MSSA and located immediately to the right of the SCC*mec* integration site.

BacLite Rapid MRSA

BacLite Rapid MRSA has been developed by Acolyte Biomedica Ltd, UK and is marketed by Bio-Stat Diagnostic Systems in the UK. The method involves a 2.5-hour selective enrichment step with oxacillin, ciprofloxacin and colistin followed by immunomagnetic separation of *S. aureus* using an anti-*S. aureus* monoclonal coupled to a magnetic bead. Separated cells are selectively lysed and detected by the novel, rapid and highly sensitive adenylate kinase (AK) bioluminescence system. Results are available in 5 hours. The assay uses conventional microbiology reagents at low volumes ensuring the cost base of the test is low. A study involving three UK hospitals based on 1387 nasal screening swabs gave a sensitivity of 93% and a specificity of 96%, a NPV of 99% and a PPV of 73%. Unlike the other four assays, this assay detects only viable organisms and highlights one of the problems associated with molecular-based assays which may detect non-viable cells.

Immunocapture-coupled PCR

This method has been developed by a research group in Switzerland and also adopts an immunomagnetic separation principle using an antibody to protein A (a *S. aureus* surface component) but does not contain a broth enrichment step. The immunocaptured *S. aureus* cells are amplified by PCR to detect the *mecA* gene and the species-specific *femA* gene of both *S. aureus* and *S. epidermidis*. Result are obtained in 6 hours. The use of this method on a medical ICU was found to reduce MRSA cross-infection on the unit substantially.

Hyplex StaphyloResist

Hyplex *Staphylo*Resist was developed by BAG-Biologische Anlaysensystem GmbH (Germany) and is marketed in the UK by The Binding Site Ltd. DNA is isolated directly from screening swabs, amplified by PCR with primers directed against *mecA* and species-specific *S. aureus* and *S. epidermidis* genes and detected by a hybridisation reaction using specific oligonucleotide probes immobilised onto microtray wells. An additional hybridisation module is available for *S. haemolyticus*. A positive result observed only in the *mecA* and the *S. aureus*-specific gene module would indicate the presence of an MRSA. However, if the *S. epidermidis* (or *S. haemolyticus*) modules were also positive, this would be interpreted as 'suspicion of MRSA' and further confirmatory tests would be required. By the 'manual' system, results are available in 4–5 hours or in < 3 hours if the automated system is used. There are no published evaluation studies to date.

GenoType MRSA Direct

This was developed by HAIN Lifescience (Germany) and is marketed in the UK by MAST. The assay involves DNA extraction direct from clinical swabs, PCR amplification using primers for *orfX* and a unique conserved region of SCC*mec*, followed by hybridisation using specific oligonucleotide probes immobilised onto membrane 'DNA Strips'. Results are available in 4 hours and unpublished evaluation studies report sensitivity and specificity of 99% and 94%, respectively, and PPV and NPV of 87% and 99.5%, respectively.

IDI MRSA

IDI MRSA was developed by Infectio Diagnostic, a Canadian company which was subsequently taken over by GeneOhm Science, recently acquired by Becton Dickinson. This assay has been validated for rapid detection of MRSA direct from nasal swabs. Theoretically, other specimens (*i.e.* wounds, blood and perineum but not axilla) could be tested but, as yet, have not been validated. Extraction of DNA directly from clinical swabs is followed by a one-step amplification and detection using real-time PCR performed with a Smart Cycler (Cepheid). Results are available within 2 hours. Like the GenoType MRSA Direct assay, this assay uses a primer in the *orfX* region but, rather than have a single primer for the SRE (SCC*mec* right extremity) region, it has primers directed to five different SRE regions located < 300 bp into SCC*mec*. The primers were designed to detect the different SCC*mec* types identified to date. The two clinical validation studies undertaken found sensitivity and specificity of 92–100% and 94–98%, respectively and a PPV of 83–95% and a NPV 97–100%. This approach appears to be very specific for *S. aureus* with no false positive results with MR-CoNS. However, 5% of MSSA tested gave false-positive results. Because this approach detects the SCC*mec* right extremity/*orfX* junction and not the *mecA* gene itself, it is possible that some MRSA may lose the *mecA* gene while retaining fragments of the SCC*mec* at the right extremity region. Furthermore, other SCC elements have been found in staphylococci which do not carry *mecA*. False-negative results have also been reported in 1% of MRSA tested suggesting that the SRE region is polymorphic and that, as yet, unrecognised sequences may be found.

Conclusions

Several national initiatives have been introduced in the last few years to combat the MRSA threat including the reporting of hospital bacteraemia rates, infection control 'Tsars', increased emphasis on hand-washing and enhanced environmental cleaning. Rapid diagnostic tests are now available which could enable the clinical microbiology laboratory to have a significant impact on the control of MRSA. All but one of the 'same-day' tests carry a large cost burden to the laboratory; however, MRSA diagnosis by '24-hour' chromogenic media and PBP2a latex appears a realistic alternative. This testing strategy would fit relatively easily into the current laboratory work-flow, has a smaller cost implication and would enable 'next-day' reporting.

Further reading
Rapid MRSA laboratory reporting

Bootsma MCJ, Diekmann O., Bonten MJM. Controlling methicillin-resistant *Staphylococcus aureus*: quantifying the effects of interventions and rapid diagnostic testing. *Proc Natl Acad Sci USA* 2006; **103**: 5620–5.

Diekema DJ, Dodgson KJ, Sigurdardottir B, Pfaller MA. Rapid detection of antimicrobial-resistant organism carriage: an unmet clinical need. *J Clin Microbiol* 2004; **42**: 2879–83.

Metan G, Zarakolu P, Unal S. Rapid detection of antibacterial resistance in emerging Gram-positive cocci. *J Hosp Infect* 2005; **61**: 93–9.

Molecular basis of methicillin resistance

Chambers HF. Methicillin resistance in staphylococci: molecular and biochemical basis and clinical implications. *Clin Microbiol Rev* 1997; **10**: 781–91.

Hiramatsu K, Katayama Y, Yuzawa H, Ito T. Molecular genetics of MRSA. *Int J Med Microbiol* 2002; **292**: 67–74.

Tomasz A, Nachman S, Leaf H. Stable classes of phenotypic expression in methicillin resistant clinical isolates of staphylococci. *Antimicrob Agents Chemother* 1991; **35**: 124–9.

Conventional MRSA laboratory reporting (2–3 day method)

Andrews J, Brenwald N, Brown DFJ, Perry J, King A, Gemmell C; for the BSAC Working Party on Susceptibility Testing. Evaluation of a 10 μg cefoxitin disc for the detection of methicillin resistance in *Staphylococcus aureus* by BSAC methodology. *J Antimicrob Chemother* 2005; **56**: 599–600.

Brown DFJ, Edwards DI, Hawkey PM *et al.*; on behalf of the Joint Working Party of the British Society for Antimicrobial Chemotherapy. Guidelines for the laboratory diagnosis and susceptibility testing of methicillin-resistant *Staphylococcus aureus* (MRSA). *J Antimicrob Chemother* 2005; **56**: 1000–18.

Next-day MRSA laboratory reporting

Fang H, Hedin G. Use of cefoxitin-based selective broth for improved detection of methicillin-resistant *Staphylococcus aureus*. *J Clin Microbiol* 2006; **44**: 592–4.

Flayhart D, Hindler JF, Bruckner DA *et al.* Multicenter evaluation of BBL CHROMagar MRSA medium for direct detection of methicillin-resistant *Staphylococcus aureus* from surveillance cultures of the anterior nares. *J Clin Microbiol* 2005; **43**: 5536–40.

Louie L, Matsumura SO, Choi E, Louie M, Simor AE. Evaluation of three rapid methods for detection of methicillin resistance in *Staphylococcus aureus*. *J Clin Microbiol* 2000; **38**: 2170–3.

Skov R, Pallesen LV, Poulsen RL, Espersen F. Evaluation of a new 3-h hybridization method for detecting the *mecA* gene in *Staphylococcus aureus* and comparison with existing genotypic and phenotypic susceptibility testing methods. *J Antimicrob Chemother* 1999; **43**: 467.

Stoakes L, Reyes R, Daniel J *et al*. Prospective comparison of a new chromogenic medium, MRSASelect, to CHROMagar MRSA and Mannitol-Salt Medium supplemented with oxacillin or cefoxitin for detection of methicillin-resistant *Staphylococcus aureus*. *J Clin Microbiol* 2006; **44**: 637–9.

Velasco D, Mar Tomas M, Cartelle M *et al*. Evaluation of different methods for detecting methicillin (oxacillin) resistance in *Staphylococcus aureus*. *J Antimicrob Chemother* 2005; **55**: 379–82.

Same-day MRSA laboratory reporting

Cuny C, Witte W. PCR for the identification of methicillin-resistant *Staphylococcus aureus* (MRSA) strains using a single primer pair specific for SCC*mec* elements and the neighbouring chromosome-borne *orfX*. *Clin Microbiol Infect* 2005; **11**: 834–7.

Francois P, Pittet D, Bento M *et al*. Rapid detection of methicillin-resistant *Staphylococcus aureus* directly from sterile or nonsterile clinical samples by a new molecular assay. *J Clin Microbiol* 2003; **41**: 254–60.

Huletsky A, Giroux R, Rossbach V *et al*. New real-time PCR assay for rapid detection of methicillin-resistant *Staphylococcus aureus* directly from specimens containing a mixture of staphylococci. *J Clin Microbiol* 2004; **42**: 1875–84.

Huletsky A, Picard FJ, Bernier M *et al*. Identification of methicillin-resistant *Staphylococcus aureus* carriage in less than 1 hour during a hospital surveillance program. *Clin Infect Dis* 2005; **40**: 976–81.

Warren DK, Liao RS, Merz LR, Eveland M, Dunne Jr WM. Detection of methicillin-resistant *Staphylococcus aureus* directly from nasal swab specimens by a real-time PCR assay. *J Clin Microbiol* 2004; **42**: 5578–81.

7. Antibiotic resistance in MRSA

Giles Edwards

Patterns of resistance
β-Lactams
Glycopeptides
Other antibiotics
Future trends

When the abbreviation MRSA began to become familiar, some clinical microbiologists thought that the letters MR might be better expanded as multi-resistant than as methicillin resistant. The significance of MRSA resulted from the difficulty in finding antibiotics to treat infections caused by it and this was often compounded by the isolates being resistant to several other antibiotics considered as possible alternatives. However, the methicillin family of penicillinase-resistant β-lactam antibiotics, especially, in the UK, flucloxacillin, predominated as first choice for the treatment of MSSA (methicillin-susceptible *Staphylococcus aureus*) infections to the extent that methicillin resistance alone necessitated a thorough reconsideration of the antibiotic treatment of *S. aureus* infections. The predominance of the use of these antibiotics resulted not only from their therapeutic effectiveness but from the rarity, at that time, of MRSA even in patients who had been treated with penicillinase-resistant β-lactams on several occasions. In contrast, the recognition, in a diagnostic laboratory, of resistance to a macrolide, usually erythromycin, in a MSSA was often an indication that the source patient had been treated with erythromycin because of a known or suspected penicillin allergy.

Nonetheless, it was recognised early that resistance to more than one class of antibiotic was normal in MRSA, most of which were being isolated from hospital patients, and that for them to be thought of as multiply resistant was useful. Multiple resistance was often defined as resistance to three or more antibiotics but that simple definition could be confusing because different laboratories often tested susceptibility to a different set of antibiotics. Some users preferred to count the number of classes of antibiotics to which resistance was detected, others counted the number of antibiotics from a particular set and yet others preferred to count the number of resistance mechanisms present. This did not, however, obscure the fact that multiresistance was indeed common in hospital isolates and that became even clearer in the late 1990s when community MRSA were first recognised; these strains are often resistant only to β-lactam antibiotics.

Patterns of resistance

> The antibiotic resistance pattern of a MRSA (its antibiogram) can change in the course of treatment by gain, or occasionally loss, of an antibiotic resistance mechanism.

This can be clinically important and it is commoner for some antibiotics than for others but its contribution to the antibiotic resistance pattern of an individual isolate is usually small relative to the resistance pattern it inherited. It follows that many strains, definitively identifiable by genotyping, can be recognised, by their antibiograms in laboratories where they are commonly seen. While a single common pattern is often easily recognisable, awareness of common variants increases the number of isolates that can be provisionally typed by phenotypic methods. Strains of the same lineage, with the same multilocus sequence type (MLST), for example, in the same geographical area will be often be identifiable like this; however, if a strain with the same MLST pattern is isolated in a different country, it cannot be recognised as confidently and, quite often, not at all. In this respect, antibiogram typing is similar to pulsed field gel electrophoresis (PFGE) typing in discriminating too finely to identify significant lineages that have diversified in different regions; geographical differences in prescribing patterns provide differing selective environments that make such effects even greater in antibiogram typing than in PFGE typing. In some situations, isolates indistinguishable by PFGE may be distinguished epidemiologically by differences in antibiogram which are due to genetic changes. Interpreting such differences in the absence of confirmatory genotypic evidence can never give a definitive answer, requires knowledge of resistance mechanisms, experience of common variations and the use of standardised testing methods but may occasionally be a useful adjunct to genotyping.

The differences in antibiograms of strains of the same lineage in different geographical settings will reflect local selection pressure and, therefore, local antibiotic use, but often in a complex way. A resistance gene may be acquired as part of a mobile genetic element transferred from another bacterium (most often also a *S. aureus*) which may also carry other genes for, perhaps, virulence, transmissibility or environmental survival. The same gene may confer resistance to several different antibiotics, usually closely related ones, and certain combinations of genes may make very successful mobile genetic elements. Many resistance genes probably confer a metabolic burden on the isolate so will only be successfully acquired in the presence of significant selective pressure but the

One of the commonly noted characteristics of community-acquired MRSA isolates is that they are less likely to be multiply resistant than hospital-type MRSA. This presumably reflects less intense use of antibiotics outside hospitals and other healthcare institutions reducing the selective advantage of multiple resistance.

acquisition of other genetic changes appears to reduce this effect. It is likely that at least some successful MRSA strains owe their success to having a greater ability than other strains to cope with the metabolic burden of accepting new genes.

The well established 'European' community MRSA (ST80-MRSA-IV), first seen in Denmark at least 10 years ago, often has several resistance markers. The isolates of this strain most often seen in Scotland are resistant to tetracycline and some aminoglycosides as well as methicillin; variants resistant to fucidin, erythromycin or ciprofloxacin are common. Similar, but rarely identical, combinations of resistances are seen in Scottish isolates of the USA300 community strain (ST8-MRSA-IV). These community strains are frequently seen in hospital patients, causing hospital-type infections, and the acquisition of multiple-resistant elements may result from spread of these strains in the hospital environment though attempts to treat recurrent or unusually unpleasant infections in the community could have a similar effect.

β-Lactams

Resistance to benzyl penicillin in *S. aureus* is caused by β-lactamase production and was recognised soon after the introduction of penicillins into clinical use. Isolates producing staphylococcal β-lactamases are also resistant to many other penicillins, including amoxycillin, and some cephalosporins. The clinical use of β-lactamase resistant penicillins, initially methicillin, was quickly followed by the detection of MRSA in 1961 but these strains did not become wide-spread for several decades. Methicillin resistance results from the production of an altered penicillin binding protein, PBP2a, a gene for which was acquired from another staphylococcal species. Antibiotics of the β-lactam group bind much less well to PBP2a than to PBP2 and, in its presence, they do not impair cell wall synthesis. This mechanism confers resistance to all generally available β-lactams but knowledge of the structure of PBP2a has allowed the development of β-lactams to which MRSA are susceptible; none are at present available for clinical use but this could change. It has also been pointed out that some of the more potent penicillinase-susceptible penicillins could have significant activity even in the presence of PBP2a and that a combination of, for example, benzyl penicillin with a β-lactamase inhibitor such as clavulanic acid might have clinically useful activity against MRSA; evidence for this from clinical trials is lacking.

Nearly all investigated MRSAs produce very similar, if not identical, PBP2a proteins but the mechanisms by which they are expressed are more variable. This reflects differences in the control genes which regulate the synthesis of PBP2a in particular and the cell wall in general. These basic mechanisms have been broadly understood for some time and in recent years more attention has been paid to the mobile resistance element, the staphylococcal chromosomal cassette (SCCmec) which carries, as well as the mecA gene and the control genes, elements which allow the cassette to be inserted into other isolates. These cassette regions have been investigated in some detail and several different PCR-based schemes have been devised for classifying them. Many of the earlier established MRSA strains contain relatively large cassettes (Types I, II and III) with additional genes, sometimes genes conferring additional antibiotic resistances, and it is assumed that these cassettes are not easily transferred between strains. The more recently recognised community isolates nearly always carry the smaller cassettes (Types IV and V) and it may be that the selection pressure that slowly led to the evolution of the smaller SCCmec cassettes played an important role in allowing the development of community MRSAs. The smaller cassettes are probably more easily acquired by established MSSA lineages and it may well be that many more MRSA lineages will emerge in the next few years. Experimental attempts have shown that, in vitro, it is very difficult to transfer even the smaller SCCmec cassette between S. aureus strains.

It has long been recognised that some reduced susceptibility to methicillin and other penicillinase resistant β-lactams is occasionally present even without the mecA gene and PBP2a. Such isolates are often referred to as borderline oxacillin-resistant S. aureus (BORSA) because the degree of resistance to oxacillin is particularly noticeable. Some such isolates have been shown to be penicillinase hyperproducers and oxacillin is more susceptible to most staphylococcal penicillinases than, for example, methicillin. Not all BORSA-like isolates are in fact hyper-penicillinase producers and other mechanisms must account for some such isolates, perhaps alterations in other penicillin binding proteins. High-level methicillin resistance, however, does not appear to occur with such mechanisms and it is widely believed that treatment with, for example, flucloxacillin at high dose is satisfactory for infections caused by such strains.

> Now that isolates strains carrying the mecA gene and mobile elements carrying it are widely dispersed, it seems unlikely that major new mechanisms of methicillin resistance will emerge.

Glycopeptides

The glycopeptides, like the β-lactams, target the cell wall but by a mechanism which excludes cross-resistance to β-lactams. Vancomycin, the first clinically available glycopeptide, was used to treat infections caused by penicillinase-producing S. aureus before penicillinase-resistant penicillins became available. The clinical efficacy and safety of antibiotics such as flucloxacillin soon restricted the use of vancomycin to treatment of infections caused by MRSA or occurring in patients with significant adverse reactions to β-lactams. A major advantage of glycopeptides was the lack of resistance to them but there was also a perception that they were less effective at curing infections or eradicating carriage.

> The use of glycopeptides only in combination with other antibiotics such as fusidic acid or gentamicin is often recommended for treatment of life-threatening infections.

Light use of vancomycin because of its perceived toxicity and the necessity for parenteral use were believed to be partly responsible for the lack of resistance in clinical isolates but difficulty in acquiring resistance also seemed important. Clinically significant, acquired glycopeptide resistance was recognised in a different Gram-positive genus (*Enterococcus*) in the 1980s and it was shown a few years later that the resistance element (the *vanA* complex) conferring high-level resistance to vancomycin and also teicoplanin could be experimentally transferred to *S. aureus* isolates which thereby acquired stable glycopeptide resistance.

The first clinical reports of glycopeptide resistance in MRSA were not, however, due to resistance transferred from enterococci but to a different mechanism which appears not to be able to confer high level resistance and is accompanied by increased thickness of the bacterial cell wall. The first such isolates were reported from Japan in 1997 and similar isolates, sometimes referred to as VISA (vancomycin-intermediate *S. aureus*), have subsequently been found in many countries, often, though not always, in patients treated with glycopeptides for prolonged periods. Infections caused by these isolates are less likely to respond to treatment with glycopeptides but much of the evidence for this is indirect. Resistance of this type may be heterogeneous (not expressed in every cell in a population though all carry the genetic element causing it) and not easily detected by techniques routinely used in diagnostic laboratories.

> In 2003, glycopeptide resistance in an MRSA and caused by the *van*A gene complex was first reported from the US and there have been three later similar reports, all from the US.

These isolates have been studied in some detail and appear to represent separate acquisition of the resistance element from enterococci. The isolates can express high-level resistance to glycopeptides but it cannot be certain that routine diagnostic laboratories would detect them. Enhanced infection control procedures seem to have prevented to spread of these isolates to identified contacts. It is, however, likely that other such isolates have been generated but not detected. If these isolates became common, it would, of course, lead to a very significant change in treatment of MRSA infections but it is very difficult to assess the probability of this happening. It took several decades for methicillin resistance to be widely accepted as a clinically important problem.

Other antibiotics

Antibiotics of many groups other than β-lactams and glycopeptides have clinically useful activity against *S. aureus*.

> For all well-established antibiotics, some acquired resistance has been found and is a potential problem in treatment of both MSSA and MRSA infections.

The wide choice of antibiotics probably reflects the clinical importance of *S. aureus* infections and the effort, therefore, put into finding therapeutic agents rather than any intrinsic susceptibility of *S. aureus*. The importance of finding new agents has been increased by the amount of resistance to older ones and in the last 5–10 years some newer antibiotics have been developed. Some of these had first been investigated some decades ago and were later brought to the market because of treatment problems caused by resistant to established agents.

> There is no good reason to believe that resistance to new agents will not spread when and where they are widely used, so it is reasonable to limit their use to where real clinical benefit is expected.

It is worth recognising that the public health benefits of restricting antibiotic use, to limit resistance, may be in conflict with the legitimate commercial interests of manufacturers and even, occasionally, with the health of an individual patient.

Several principles can help prescribers, and those who advise them, to limit the development of resistance. The use of combination therapy, particularly when antibiotics known to give rise to resistance easily are being used, can reasonably be expected to make the emergence of resistant isolates less likely and knowing the antibiotic susceptibility of strains causing individual infections allows this to be done more effectively. Where the susceptibility of individual isolates cannot be tested, then knowledge of local resistance patterns can be helpful. For antibiotics known to give rise to resistance easily, then short courses of, perhaps, 5 days, guided by clinical response may be helpful. In the UK, it is unusual for even a hospital-acquired MRSA not to be susceptible to at least two orally available antibiotics. It has occasionally been suggested that, as many S. aureus infections are minor and self-limiting, apparently trivial infections should not be treated with antibiotics; indeed, many are not but it must be recognised that if this became deliberate practice then, occasionally, significant infections would become life-threatening. Failed attempts to eradicate MRSA carriage may be an important factor in selecting resistant strains, so attempts to eliminate carriage should be restricted to patients who are likely to benefit, take into account the likelihood of acquisition of a replacement strain, follow appropriate protocols and only be repeated after due consideration.

There follows a brief account of relevant aspects of a number of antibiotics.

Macrolides and clindamycin

For many years, erythromycin has been a common choice for treatment of MSSA infections in patients for whom adverse reactions to β-lactams are anticipated. Perhaps as a result of this, erythromycin resistance is very common in MRSAs. In the UK, almost all EMRSA-16 isolates are resistant and about 80% of EMRSA-15 isolates. The occasional erythromycin sensitive isolate of EMRSA-15 probably results from the loss of a plasmid and it may be that many EMRSA-15 populations are a mixture of resistant and susceptible cells. Erythromycin is, therefore, rarely useful for treatment of MRSA infections. Not all erythromycin resistance is plasmid borne and there are several different mechanisms of resistance; cross resistance to other macrolides such as clarithromycin and azithromycin is normal. The commonest resistance mechanism in UK strains is a ribosomal modification known as MLS resistance (because it confers resistance to macrolides, lincosamides and streptogramins). Strains of this kind may be susceptible to clindamycin (a lincosamide) on routine testing but erythromycin can induce clindamycin resistance (sometimes referred to as dissociated resistance) in such strains and constitutively clindamycin resistant variants are readily produced. In general, clindamycin should not be used, at least as sole agent, to treat erythromycin resistant S. aureus, unless the resistance is known not to be of the MLS type.

Aminoglycosides

Aminoglycosides, such as gentamicin and amikacin, act against ribosomes, and are active against both Gram-negative and Gram-positive organisms. They have reputation for synergy with some other antibiotics and for toxicity. They are not well absorbed orally and not secreted usefully into the CSF. Some are available in topical formulations. This combination of features makes them a valuable part of the treatment of life-threatening infections and limited use of this kind might be expected to result in resistance being rare. Aminoglycoside resistance is, however, fairly common in hospital MRSAs and can be due to several different mechanisms. Resistance in staphylococci is often due to the presence of one of a fairly small number of aminoglycoside modifying enzymes, often encoded as one of a number of resistance genes on a mobile genetic element. Different enzymes confer resistance to different combinations of aminoglycosides and individual enzymes can often be identified from the resistance pattern though it is not unusual for an isolate to have genes for more than one enzyme. Particular enzymes may be commonly seen in a particular strain and one particular enzyme is seen in two quite distinct community-type MRSA strains in Scotland (ST8-MRSA-IV and ST80-MRSA-IV) but only rarely in hospital-type MRSA; the reason for this is unclear.

Tetracyclines

Before the emergence of EMRSA-15 and EMRSA-16 in the UK, tetracycline resistance was so common as to be used in some diagnostic laboratories as a marker for methicillin resistance on screening plates. Few hospital isolates (< 10%) are now resistant to tetracycline and, in combination with other oral agents, tetracyclines such as doxycycline can be therapeutically useful if susceptibility has been demonstrated. When the isolates of the older strains are encountered, they are usually still tetracycline resistant and many, though not all, Scottish isolates of the ST80-MRSA-IV lineage are tetracycline resistant. Several different resistance mechanisms are recognised and resistance genes have been recognised on different transferable resistance elements in combinations with genes conferring resistance to antibiotics such as aminoglycosides and mupirocin. Tetracycline resistance may be being maintained in MRSA populations, despite the reduction in tetracycline use, partly by selection for resistance to other antibiotics.

Fluoroquinolones

In contrast to tetracycline resistance, ciprofloxacin resistance is extremely common in hospital strains of MRSA but rarer in community strains and in MSSA. Some selective media used by diagnostic laboratories for MRSA screening contain ciprofloxacin as a selective agent. Ciprofloxacin resistance appears to be fairly easily acquired in association with therapeutic use and results from modification of the target enzyme. Ciprofloxacin-resistant isolates usually have reduced susceptibility to other fluoroquinolones but the isolates may have minimal inhibitory concentrations (MICs) within the susceptible range for, for example, moxifloxacin.

Quinolones are useful agents for the treatment of infections caused by susceptible isolates though they cannot be recommended for use without specific susceptible testing. Even for susceptible isolates, combination therapy with another agent is advisable for serious infections.

Rifampicin

Resistance to rifampicin is easily detected in the laboratory and appears to be easily acquired during treatment. Rifampicin is quite widely used in combination with other agents, such as glycopeptides, for treatment of serious MRSA infections but susceptibility must be demonstrated before use and, if prolonged treatment is used, continued susceptibility should be monitored. The frequency of resistance found depends upon the amount of local use.

Sodium fusidate

Sodium fusidate has good activity against *S. aureus* but is rarely useful for treating infections caused by other bacteria. As with rifampicin, isolates readily acquire resistance during treatment and against serious infection the two antibiotics are often used in similar ways. However, sodium fusidate is also available in topical formulations and is widely used, especially outside hospitals, for superficial infections. This may account for resistance being quite common in community strains, especially in those (MRSA and MSSA) producing exfoliative toxins and, therefore, needing repeated treatment in the community.

Trimethoprim

Trimethoprim, even outside the combination (cotrimoxazole) with sulphamethoxazole, has good activity against isolates of *S. aureus* which have not acquired resistance but resistance is fairly easily acquired and may be difficult to detect confidently in the laboratory. In addition, the laboratory breakpoints required to guide treatment regimens are not well established. Nonetheless, trimethoprim is quite widely used in combination treatment with agents such as sodium fusidate or tetracyclines.

Mupirocin

Mupirocin is only available as a topical agent and resistance in MRSA was seen soon after it became widely used. Resistance shown in the laboratory can be grouped into two categories – high level (MIC > 1024 mg/l) and low level (MIC 32–64 mg/l); it results from modification of the target enzyme (isoleucyl tRNA synthetase). Low-level resistance is of doubtful clinical significance but high-level resistance, usually plasmid borne and transferable, is associated with treatment failure. Most strains seem to be able to acquire high-level resistance and its frequency depends on local usage of mupirocin, or of other antibiotics for which resistance genes are found on the same transferable genetic element.

Newer agents

Among the antibiotics in which there has been recently increased interest are quinupristin–dalfopristin (a combination of streptogramins), linezolid (an oxazolidinone) and daptomycin (a cyclic lipopeptide). Resistance to all these antibiotics is possible but they have not yet been used widely enough to predict how significant a problem resistance will become.

Future trends

As illustrated above, the great majority of MRSA isolates are susceptible to several available antibiotics but a great deal of attention is understandably paid to the small number of isolates which are susceptible to very few antibiotics. It is certainly possible that, in the presence of unrestricted antibiotic use, such strain could become more and more common in hospitals but the selective pressure in the community is very different because the intensity of antibiotic use is much lower. Certainly, the development of new antibiotics and experience in their use is important to the treatment of MRSA infections in hospitals; however, in the community, knowledge of the susceptibility of individual isolates, the use of already available antibiotics and the avoidance of blind therapy may be as important. The use of blind therapy has been a mainstay of community treatment because of the relative inaccessibility of laboratory support; the use of surveillance data could help.

In many UK hospitals, several different MRSA strains, with different sensitivity patterns are endemic and the selection pressure of antibiotic use is as likely to lead to acquisition of a replacement strain as to acquisition of a new resistance mechanism. In this environment, limiting the spread of isolates by good infection control practice is just as important to the control of antibiotic resistance as is control of antibiotic use. In the community, where, at present, other multiply resistant isolates are less likely to be found and preventing the transmission of bacteria from person to person is even more difficult, the balance may shift more towards control of antibiotic use.

Further reading

Appelbaum PC. The emergence of vancomycin-intermediate and vancomycin-resistant *Staphylococcus aureus*. *Clin Microbiol Infect* 2006; **12 (Suppl 1)**: 16–23.

Kucers A, Crowe SM, Grayson ML, Hoy J. *The Use of Antibiotics*. Oxford: Butterworth Heinemann, 1997 [A text giving well-referenced information on resistance mechanism to established antibiotics].

Schito GC. The importance of the development of antibiotic resistance in *Staphylococcus aureus*. *Clin Microbiol Infect* 2006; **12 (Suppl 1)**: 3–8.

8. Clinical features of community-acquired MRSA

Tristan Ferry, Jerome Etienne

CA-MRSA skin and soft tissue infections

CA-MRSA pulmonary infections

CA-MRSA bone and joint infections

Other CA-MRSA organ infections

CA-MRSA bacteraemia and
   disseminated infections

CA-MRSA septic shock and purpura
   fulminans

Diagnosis of CA-MRSA infections

General recommendations for patients
   with CA-MRSA infections

The overall percentage of *Staphylococcus aureus* isolates expressing methicillin resistance has increased significantly in the community during the past two decades, but two main types of MRSA circulate in the community:

1. Hospital-derived strains carried into the community and spread by person-to-person contact. These strains are similar to those spreading in the hospitals. These strains tend to infect old patients with a median age over 65 years, who usually have underlying diseases (diabetes mellitus, cancer, chronic skin disease, surgical incisions, *etc.*), and/or in-dwelling urinary tract or intravascular devices, and/or a history of hospitalisation, and/or are under haemodialysis. Such MRSA infections seen in the community can be acquired either directly in hospitals or long-term care facilities during a previous stay, or indirectly by contact with an MRSA carrier such as a family member working in a hospital, or a healthcare worker such as a community nurse.

2. Strains arising *de novo* in the community and infecting patients with none of the above established risk factors. These strains tend to infect children and young healthy adults. They differ from the strains transmitted within hospitals, as they frequently harbour specific virulence factors such as the Panton-Valentine leukocidin (PVL) genes. PVL is a potent necrotising toxin, able to lyse the host cell membrane, especially human polymorphonuclear neutrophils, monocytes and macrophages.

Community-acquired MRSA (CA-MRSA) infections described in this chapter correspond to those associated with MRSA strains that have emerged recently (by the early 1990s) *de novo* in the community and frequently containing the PVL genes.

> These CA-MRSA infections have emerged world-wide and are associated with a limited number of clones that are highly epidemic in the community.

Such infections are becoming increasingly common, especially in certain US states. In Europe, the prevalence is low but is gradually increasing. Outbreaks of CA-MRSA infections, especially of skin and soft tissue infections have been described among members of 'closed populations', such as competitive athletes, jail inmates, military recruits, men who have sex with men, and children in schools or in child care-centres.

> CA-MRSA is mainly transmitted from man-to-man by direct skin-to-skin contact, or indirectly through contact by touching objects (*e.g.* towels, sheets, linen, pillows, wound dressings, clothes, workout areas, sports equipment) contaminated by the infected skin of a person with MRSA.

Most CA-MRSA infections are represented by superficial skin and soft tissue infections. These infections are usually non-severe, although frequently requiring incision and surgical drainage. Deep-seated infections associated with CA-MRSA (*e.g.* necrotising pneumonia) are rare, but are extremely severe and life-threatening. Finally, the progressive spread of these highly epidemic MRSA clones in the community could be associated in the future with a more frequent recognition of such severe clinical syndromes associated with the production of PVL by *S. aureus*.

CA-MRSA skin and soft tissue infections

The *S. aureus* skin infections are considered 'primary' in patients with no pre-existing skin lesion, and 'secondary' in other cases. CA-MRSA causes predominantly primary skin and soft tissue infections that account for 95% of these infections.

The primary lesion of the skin caused by CA-MRSA is due to a direct invasion and tissue destruction by the strain which is enhanced by the production of PVL.

> Furunculosis is the most frequently reported initial presentation of CA-MRSA infection and is usually the first step before the skin abscess formation.

The elemental furuncle lesion is characterised by a painful red nodule with a central pustule. Furuncles occur usually on the lower extremities. At infection onset, the lesion can look minimal and patients often complain of a mosquito or an insect bite. Furuncles due to CA-MRSA can be multiple, tend to evolve with intense erythema around the lesions (which may reflect strong inflammation caused by polymorphonuclear cells and capillary dilation due to the production of PVL). Other primary necrotic lesions such as deep punched-out ulcers with black eschars have also been described and any primary lesion can be associated with tender fluctuant local lymph nodes or overlying cellulitis. The striking features of CA-MRSA skin infection are necrosis and pus formation, and the frequent progression to the formation of abscesses which usually necessitate surgical treatment.

Skin or soft-tissue abscesses due to CA-MRSA can be severe by their localisation or by the intensity of the inflammatory lesion. When localised on the face, CA-MRSA abscesses can lead to orbital cellulitis, pansinusitis and cavernous sinus thrombosis. When localised on the hand, the infection can lead to the destruction of tendons. Recently, some cases of pyomyositis due to CA-MRSA have been described. Pyomyositis is a pyogenic infection of a skeletal muscle rarely reported in temperate climates and usually due to methicillin-susceptible *S. aureus*. Pyomyositis due to CA-MRSA occurred a few weeks after the surgical drainage of a furuncle in the underlying muscle or in a distinct site by haematogenous spread.

Necrotising fasciitis due to CA-MRSA is also an emerging severe infection. It is a severe, soft-tissue infection characterised by wide-spread fascial necrosis, exceptionally associated with *S. aureus* monomicrobial infection. Necrotising fasciitis due to CA-MRSA has been described in patients for whom the pre-operative diagnosis was skin or soft-tissue abscesses; most had documented co-existing conditions (injection-drug abuse, diabetes or chronic hepatitis C). These rapidly progressive cases of necrotising fasciitis are clinically indistinguishable from those caused by the group A streptococci.

Cases of folliculitis and impetigo associated with CA-MRSA have been described. CA-MRSA bullous impetigo (sometimes scabby impetigo) is a localised skin infection associated with the production of an exfoliative toxin that enhances skin damage by cleaving the epithelium at the level of zona granulosa.

CA-MRSA pulmonary infections

Severe necrotising pneumonia due to CA-MRSA has occasionally been described mostly in previously healthy children and teenagers. This disease is strongly associated with *S. aureus* strains producing PVL. PVL-positive CA-MRSA can infect lungs via the respiratory tract mainly after a flu-like respiratory infection or via the bloodstream. Influenza virus is known to increase respiratory colonisation by *S. aureus* and to impair ciliary function (and, therefore, the clearance of *S. aureus*). In the classic scenario of PVL-associated necrotising pneumonia, a patient develops a flu-like respiratory illness and then, after few days, deteriorates rapidly with fever and dyspnoea. The syndrome is characterised by high fever, haemoptysis, hypotension, leukopenia, and multilobular alveolar infiltrates with pleural effusion that, unlike nosocomial MRSA pneumonias, usually progress into abscesses and empyema. Blood cultures are positive for *S. aureus* in half of the cases. A rapid progression to septic shock and acute respiratory distress syndrome is the rule. The mortality is extremely high (50–75%). Autopsy shows diffuse bilateral necrotic and haemorrhagic pneumonia, whereas lung computed tomography shows destruction of the parenchyma.

Various pulmonary manifestations can also occur via the bloodstream in patients with an extra-lung primary invasive CA-MRSA infection. This metastatic pulmonary disease can be seen in patients with bone and joint infection. Radiographic findings often reveal single or multiple lobar alveolar infiltrates, a pneumonia with pneumotaceles, a lung abscess, an empyema or multiple nodular densities suggestive of septic emboli.

CA-MRSA bone and joint infections

Cases of osteomyelitis and septic arthritis caused by CA-MRSA have been reported, mainly in children. The clinical characteristics of these infections are not well defined, but these infections are usually severe. The presence of PVL genes is associated with an increased likelihood of complications and more frequent development of chronic osteomyelitis. Repetitive trips to the operating room for irrigation and debridement of osteomyelitis are often required. Bone or joint infections due to

CA-MRSA have also been reported in adults and most were associated with bacteraemia and disseminated infection. The occurrence of deep venous thrombosis in association with staphylococcal osteomyelitis may have a role in the dissemination of CA-MRSA by causing septic pulmonary emboli.

Other CA-MRSA organ infections

Organ abscesses involving, for example, the prostate or a kidney have been described as the primary diagnosis of a CA-MRSA infection. They are usually associated with haematogenous spread of CA-MRSA and disseminated infection.

CA-MRSA bacteraemia and disseminated infections

Bacteraemia during CA-MRSA infections may be associated with a disseminated infection characterised by multiple abscesses within lung, muscle and bone infections. Bacteraemia occurs frequently during necrotising pneumonia and metastatic pulmonary infections have also become increasingly apparent in patients with bone and joint infection. The evidence of multiple disseminated abscesses in a patient with MRSA bacteraemia is highly likely to be due to a PVL-positive strain.

Endocarditis due to CA-MRSA is infrequent but vegetations on cardiac valves are sometimes discovered in those cases of disseminated infections. As a result, evaluation of all patients for endocarditis is recommended when blood cultures are positive for *S. aureus*.

CA-MRSA septic shock and purpura fulminans

Septic shock and multi-organ dysfunction occur mainly during necrotising pneumonia and disseminated cases of CA-MRSA infections. Purpura fulminans and the Waterhouse-Friderichsen syndrome (characterised by bilateral adrenal haemorrhage), which usually occur during fulminant meningococcaemia, have recently been described during CA-MRSA septic shock.

Diagnosis of CA-MRSA infections

The diagnosis of MRSA should be suggested if the infection persists or progresses during treatment that was directed toward methicillin-susceptible *S. aureus*. If a bacterial culture was not performed at the initial visit or if surgical intervention is necessary, there is a need to consider sending a culture to establish the identity and antibiotic sensitivity of the pathogenic bacteria.

> CA-MRSA isolates are typically sensitive to a wide variety of non-β-lactam antibiotics including trimethoprim-sulfamethoxazole, minocycline, fluoroquinolones, vancomyin, linezolid, quinupristin-dalfopristin, and daptomycin.

The delayed use of effective antibiotics may contribute to higher rates of disability and death. Vancomycin can be used in serious or life-threatening infections suspected to be MRSA.

Between 36–92% of patients with CA-MRSA skin infections require incision and drainage of their skin lesion.

General recommendations for patients with CA-MRSA infections

As CA-MRSA is easily transmitted, patients with soft-tissue infections should be counselled on the importance of hand hygiene, not sharing personal items such as towels, and appropriate wound care. Preventing transmission of MRSA to other individuals, such as family members and team-mates, is also important.

> Patients with CA-MRSA skin infections should maximise personal hygiene with particular attention toward hand-washing.

Potentially contaminated items from the environment (athletic equipment, shaving razors, and cloth products that have been in contact with infected skin, such as towels and clothing), should be either cleaned or removed.

Further reading

Cohen PR, Kurzrock R. Community-acquired methicillin-resistant *Staphylococcus aureus* skin infection: an emerging clinical problem. *J Am Acad Dermatol* 2004; **50**: 277–80.

Crum NF. The emergence of severe, community-acquired methicillin-resistant *Staphylococcus aureus* infections. *Scand J Infect Dis* 2005; **37**: 651–6.

Fagan SP, Berger DH, Rahwan K *et al*. Spider bites presenting with methicillin-resistant *Staphylococcus aureus* soft tissue infection require early aggressive treatment. *Surg Infect* 2003; **4**: 311–5.

Gillet Y, Issartel B, Vanhems P *et al*. Association between *Staphylococcus aureus* strains carrying gene for Panton-Valentine leukocidin and highly lethal necrotising pneumonia in young immunocompetent patients. *Lancet* 2002; **359**: 753–9.

Gonzalez BE, Hulten KG, Dishop MK *et al*. Pulmonary manifestations in children with invasive community-acquired *Staphylococcus aureus* infection. *Clin Infect Dis* 2005; **41**: 583–90.

Gonzalez BE, Martinez-Aguilar G, Hulten KG et al. Severe staphylococcal sepsis in adolescents in the era of community-acquired methicillin-resistant *Staphylococcus aureus*. *Pediatrics* 2005; **115**: 642–8.

Issartel B, Tristan A, Lechevallier S *et al*. Frequent carriage of Panton-Valentine leucocidin genes by *Staphylococcus aureus* isolates from surgically drained abscesses. *J Clin Microbiol* 2005; **43**: 3203–7.

Miller LG, Perdreau-Remington F, Rieg G *et al*. Necrotizing fasciitis caused by community-associated methicillin-resistant *Staphylococcus aureus* in Los Angeles. *N Engl J Med* 2005; **352**: 1445–53.

Rutar T, Zwick OM, Cockerham KP *et al*. Bilateral blindness from orbital cellulitis caused by community-acquired methicillin-resistant *Staphylococcus aureus*. *Am J Ophthalmol* 2005; **140**: 740–2.

Zetola N, Francis JS, Nuermberger EL *et al*. Community-acquired meticillin-resistant *Staphylococcus aureus*: an emerging threat. *Lancet Infect Dis* 2005; **5**: 275–86.

9. Clinical presentation of MRSA infections

Hisham Ziglam, Dilip Nathwani

Colonisation and infection

Infections associated with MRSA

Skin and soft-tissue infection

MRSA bacteraemia

MRSA endocarditis

MRSA and bone infection

Hospital/ventilator acquired pneumonia

MRSA and postoperative infections

Conclusions

Staphylococcus aureus is a virulent pathogen that causes human infections ranging from asymptomatic colonisation to local, often supparative, infections such as skin and soft-tissue infections, and severe systemic infections, such as endovascular infections.

> A recent global comprehensive international survey of clinical isolates found that *S. aureus* accounted for 22% of all bloodstream infections, 39% of all skin and soft-tissue infections and 23.2% of lower respiratory tract infections.[1]

Hospital-acquired infection is classically defined as infection not present or incubating at the time of admission, and is usually defined operationally as infection occurring more than 48 hours after admission.[2] Indeed, *S. aureus* infections are leading causes of nosocomial infections including surgical wound infections (28%) and pneumonia (28%).[3] On the other hand, in the community they are the commonest cause of osteomyelitis (50–70%)

and a major cause of bacteraemia (15–23.5%) and endocarditis.[4] The burden of these infections, and the percentage due to MRSA, in US hospitals has recently been estimated. *S. aureus* infection accounted for 0.8% of all US in-patient diagnosis between 2000 and 2001 and represented an average of 3 times length of stay and hospital charges and 5 times the risk of hospital death compared with in-patients without infection.[5] From 1999 to 2000, an estimated 125,969 hospitalisations were due to MRSA of which 31,440 were septicaemia and 29,823 pneumonia.[6] Whilst these data represent a high burden of MSSA and MRSA infections causing nosocomial and community-onset infections, to our knowledge the clinical presentations of MRSA infections do not appear to differ from those of MSSA infections[7] although there is controversy around overall increased virulence and mortality. Two meta-analyses[8,9] suggest that MRSA infections are associated with greater overall mortality (~ 2-fold) although, until a prospective study links risk factors to the individual patients, we cannot definitively conclude that MRSA infections are intrinsically more lethal than MSSA infections.

> The clinical presentations of MRSA infections do not appear to differ from those of MSSA infections.

Colonisation and infection

Several factors may contribute to increased risk for MSSA and MRSA colonisation and subsequent infection (Table 9.1).

> Humans are natural reservoirs of *S. aureus* with 30–50% of healthy adults colonised and 10–20% persistently colonised.

Apart from classical risk factors such as type 1 diabetes, intravenous drug misuse, haemodialysis, and AIDS, other common risk

Table 9.1
Risk factors associated with MRSA

- Diabetes mellitus
- Male gender
- Length of hospitalisation
- Stay in an ICU
- Exposure to colonised or infected patient
- Intravenous drug use
- Haemodialysis
- Major surgical procedures
- Immunocompromised conditions
  - AIDS
  - Quantitative defect in leukocyte function
  - Qualitative defect in leukocyte function (e.g. Chediak-Higashi syndrome, chronic granulomatous disease, Job's syndrome)
- History of long-term or frequent antibiotic use
- Invasive lines or tube (intravenous, urinary catheters
- Increased age (elderly)
- History of multiple hospitalisations or procedures
- Infections/colonisation at other sites
- Morbid obesity
- Orthopaedic implant surgery
- Long-term in-patient stay

factors include healthcare contact, longer duration of hospitalisation,[10,11] severe underlying disease, intravascular catheter infection, wound infection, hospitalisation in ICU, and prior antibiotic therapy. These factors are similar across a range of bacteria and seem to relate to the patient's direct or indirect exposure to hospitals.[12]

> As up to 80% of cases of *S. aureus* bacteraemia are due to the strain isolated in the anterior nares of the patient, screening of patients with risk factors and subsequent eradication of carriage would seem reasonable to prevent infection.

Colonisation with MRSA is particularly linked to older age, receipt of antimicrobials within the previous year (duration and type of antibiotic also appears to influence this), previous hospitalisation within 3 years, and a known history of previous MRSA.[13]

> Carriage of MRSA appears also to be more closely associated with invasive infection than MSSA. For example, Pujol *et al.*[14] showed that nasal carriage of MRSA in ICU patients was associated with an MRSA bacteraemia rate of 38% – 4-fold higher than MSSA.

Whilst carriage acts as the principal reservoir for infection to the patient and transmission of infection to other patients, it has been suggested that this knowledge, in the absence of clinical differentiating factors and rapid microbiology, may be valuable in the overall clinical decision-making process determining appropriate empiric therapy in critically unwell patients with *S. aureus* infections.

Community-acquired MRSA (CA-MRSA) has emerged as a cause of skin infections in the community (up to 77% of all infections). Other infections included bacteraemia, bone and joint infections (6%) and pneumonia, often severe and fatal (2%). Criteria for determining the likelihood of a strain being CA-MRSA are provided in Table 9.2,[15] although the value of such case definitions in clinical practice has not been validated. Clinicians should now consider CA-MRSA as a potential pathogen in patients with suspected *S. aureus* infections in the community setting. A significant proportion

Table 9.2
Criteria of people who likely have community-acquired MRSA (CA-MRSA) infections

- Diagnosis of MRSA was made in the out-patient setting or by a culture positive for MRSA within 48 hours after admission to the hospital
- The patient has no medical history of MRSA infection or colonisation.
- The patient has no medical history in the past year of:
  - Hospitalisation
  - Admission to a nursing home or hospice
  - Dialysis
  - Surgery
- The patient has no permanent in-dwelling catheters or medical devices that pass through the skin into the body

(23%) of patients in this large cohort were hospitalised, reflecting their overall severity.[15] Although true CA-MRSA infections have emerged as a significant public health problem, it is difficult to determine what the effect of these infections will have on the incidence of MRSA infections among hospitalised patients. The majority of patients who have MRSA infection apparently from the community have usually had recent hospital contact. In a recent study from Oxford, UK, 91% of those with MRSA bacteraemia had been in hospital a median time of 46 days earlier and 31% had prior intensive exposure to renal or haematology/oncology wards.[16]

Infections associated with MRSA

S. aureus is responsible for significant proportions of both community-acquired and nosocomial infections (Table 9.3). Until recently, most MRSA infections have occurred in hospitalised patients and nosocomial MRSA infection rates have varied widely from hospital to hospital and from country to country in Europe.[17]

Skin and soft-tissue infection

Skin and soft-tissue infections are clearly the most common clinical MRSA infection.

Staphylococcal skin infections may be differentiated clinically from Group A streptococcal skin infection by the presence of bullae and the absence of systemic symptoms.

Staphylococcal abscesses may be accompanied by high fever and chills. With staphylococcal cellulitis, chills are not prominent, in contrast with streptococcal cellulitis.

The risk of postoperative wound infection is not the same for all patients. The traditional infection risk protocol, first developed in the early 1960s, divided surgical procedures into 4 classes – clean (Class I); clean-contaminated (Class II); contaminated (Class III); and dirty (Class IV) – each with a different risk of infection. Later studies identified ranges of risk for each class: clean (1–5% infection risk), clean-contaminated (3–11%), contaminated (10–17%), and dirty (27%).[18] Nasal carriage of *S. aureus* was first identified as a risk factor for auto-infection of surgical wounds in the late 1950s.

Recent studies have confirmed the importance of pre-operative *S. aureus* carriage in causing postoperative wound infections. Among patients who acquired *S. aureus* infections and for whom paired isolates were available, 84.6% of the *S. aureus* surgical site infections were caused by the strains the patients carried pre-operatively.

MRSA bacteraemia

Nosocomial bloodstream infections require special consideration since they are frequent (*e.g.* 12% of all nosocomial infections reported in a study on more than 10,000 European intensive care patients[19]) and carry significant

Table 9.3
Relative frequency of *S. aureus* as a cause of selected infection

Infection type	Community-acquired (n = 131)	Healthcare-acquired (n = 937)
Skin/soft tissue	98 (75%)	343 (37%)
Otitis media/externa	9 (7%)	11 (1%)
Respiratory tract	8 (6%)	205 (22%)
Bloodstream	5 (4%)	83 (9%)
Urinary tract	1 (1%)	185 (20%)
Others	10 (8%)	110 (12%)

Adapted from Naimi *et al.*[44]

attributable mortality (4–30%) and costs (US$ 4000–40,000).[20] Intravascular catheter related infections are the primary cause of nosocomial bacteraemia[20] and it has been shown that the mortality rate attributed to catheter-related *S. aureus* bacteraemia (8.2%) significantly exceeds the rates for other pathogens.[21]

> *S. aureus* bloodstream infections frequently cause metastatic infections of numerous sites, including heart valves, bones, joints, and eyes.[22]

A few case series have looked at the impact of methicillin resistance on outcome in bacteraemic patients, with conflicting results. Harbarth *et al.*[23] reported that methicillin resistance in patients with *S. aureus* bacteraemia had no significant impact on patient outcome as measured by in-hospital mortality rate after adjustment was made for the severity of underlying diseases. This finding was supported by a recent analysis by Cosgrove *et al.*[24] who found no difference in mortality between MRSA and MSSA bacteraemia but significant increase in length of hospital stay and charges.

Patients with staphylococcal bacteraemia usually have a demonstrable focus of infection involving the skin/soft tissues or emanating from a bone/joint infection. In the absence of a recognisable focus for staphylococcal bacteraemia, an endovascular infection (*e.g.* endocarditis) should be considered.[25] In patients with *S. aureus* bacteraemia, Lodise *et al.*[26] predicted the likelihood of MRSA in a particular patient with infective endocarditis by a clinical decision rule. The presence of hospitalisation, recent long duration of hospital stay, recent course of antibiotics and the presence of a decubitus ulcer increase the likelihood of the infection being MRSA. These kind of clinical decision rules may allow clinicians to predict early appropriate empiric therapy.[26]

MRSA endocarditis

Infective endocarditis was an invariably fatal infection before the availability of antimicrobials. Even after the introduction of antibiotic therapy and valve replacement, the reported early mortality rate of infective endocarditis remains high (16–31%), and the mortality rate after 5–10 years' follow-up ranges from 25% to 50%.[27] *S. aureus* is the most frequent micro-organism isolated from the blood, carries the worst prognosis and has a high prevalence of embolic episodes and complications.[28] MRSA acts as a significant cause of infective endocarditis internationally, accounting for almost 40% of the infective endocarditis caused by *S. aureus* in certain regions.

> About 20% of patients with MRSA infective endocarditis develop infection in the absence of identifiable healthcare contact. This finding might suggest that community-acquired MRSA may be an emerging cause of infective endocarditis in many regions of the world.

The clinical differentiation of *S. aureus* bacteraemia from infective endocarditis has long been a vexing problem for clinicians and has obvious therapeutic and prognostic implications. In the absence of typical Oslerian manifestations (such as changing murmur, splenomegaly, embolic lesions), the clinical diagnosis of infective endocarditis among patients with *S. aureus* bacteraemia can be challenging. Nolan *et al.*[29] reported three useful bedside criteria for predicting the presence of infective endocarditis in patients with *S. aureus* bacteraemia: (i) community acquisition; (ii) no apparent primary focus; and (iii) the occurrence of metastatic foci. An increased incidence of endocarditis has also been observed in populations with a large proportion of intravenous drug users[30] or with underlying valvular heart disease, or prior endocarditis. Chang and colleagues[31–33] revealed that MRSA endocarditis was more likely to be hospital acquired (including patients on haemodialysis), while MSSA endocarditis was more likely to be community acquired. It has been recognised that patients with MRSA endocarditis had a longer duration of fever after active antibiotic therapy was initiated, were significantly more likely to have persistent bacteraemia, and had a higher incidence of renal insufficiency. It is interesting to find that patients with healthcare-associated *S. aureus* infective endocarditis had higher rates of in-hospital mortality than did patients with community-acquired *S. aureus* infective endocarditis.[31–33] The course is frequently fulminant when it involves the mitral or aortic valve, with wide-spread metastatic infection to distant organs (*i.e.* the central nervous system, the heart, spleen, lungs, kidneys and joints) and results in death in approximately 40% of patients; the mortality rate often exceeds 50% in patients over 50 years of age.[34]

MRSA and bone infection

Despite the increasing importance of MRSA as a nosocomial and community pathogen, little is known about the clinical characteristics of MRSA septic arthritis. In European studies,[35,36] 6–8% of cases of septic arthritis were due to MRSA. The clinical presentation of MRSA septic arthritis or osteomyelitis is indistinguishable from similar infections caused by other organisms. However, a recent study revealed that MRSA septic arthritis was more commonly associated with fever, leukocytosis, bacteraemia and has a tendency to involve more than one joint compared with non-MRSA septic arthritis.[37] Vertebral osteomyelitis is also a common, and often unrecognised, complication of *S. aureus* bacteraemia.[38] Elderly patients may frequently develop a paravertebral abscess following staphylococcal bacteraemia as the initial manifestation of vertebral osteomyelitis.[38] There is no data about these infections specific to MRSA.

Prosthetic joint infections, usually involving the hip or knee, are most often caused by strains of coagulase-negative staphylococci. However, *S. aureus* is second only to the coagulase-negative staphylococci as an important pathogen in prosthetic joint infections. MRSA may affect knee or hip prostheses.

> In contrast with low virulence organisms (*e.g.* the coagulase-negative staphylococci), *S. aureus* is more likely to present as acute prosthetic joint infection.[39]

MRSA infections are also now a leading cause of cardiothoracic sternotomy site infections, often with sternal bone osteomyelitis.[40]

Hospital/ventilator acquired pneumonia

Nosocomial pneumonia is currently the second most common hospital infection and is the leading cause of death from hospital-acquired infections. The incidence of acquiring nosocomial pneumonia ranges from 7.8% to 68.0%, and is influenced by the duration of hospital and ICU stay, the specific diagnostic method used for pathogen detection, and the patient population studied. The rate of nosocomial pneumonia secondary to *S. aureus* has increased steadily over the past two decades. Ventilator-associated pneumonia (VAP) is the leading nosocomial infection in the ICU. MRSA pneumonias are common in patients with prolonged intubation periods, prior use of antibiotics within a previous 90-day period, those who have been hospitalised for more that 5 days and where there is a high prevalence of MRSA within the hospital.

> MRSA pneumonia does not appear to present clinically different to MSSA pneumonia but success despite treatment with glycopeptides is only in the region of ~50%.[41]

The suspicion of a new episode of VAP has to be established in all intubated patients with clinical signs of sepsis. Once a patient develops fever and leukocytosis, the physicians must promptly identify the source of infection in order to start adequate empiric antibiotic therapy, based on risk factors for resistance, so as to ensure the most optimal outcome. This therapy ought to be changed in light of the results of investigations.

MRSA and postoperative infections

Two prospective multicentre audits were performed to examine graft infections in Britain and Ireland with particular reference to outcome associated with MRSA infection (Table 9.4).

Table 9.4

Core risk factors for MRSA colonisation/infection in postoperative surgical patients

Patient-related
- Known colonisation
- Open, chronic skin wound or breakage
- Obesity
- End-stage renal disease, diabetes mellitus, liver failure or spinal injury

Treatment-related
- Previous antibiotic therapy
- Hospital stay > 2 weeks
- Invasive procedure or intravenous catheterisation especially central venous lines
- Prolonged mechanical ventilation

Environment
- Long-term care facility
- Prolonged hospitalisation, especially in high-risk areas such as high dependency

Adapted from Solomkin et al.[45]

MRSA was the commonest single organism cultured in patients with complex wound and graft infections after vascular surgery and contributed towards an increased risk of adverse outcome and prolonged hospital stay.[42]

The clinical presentation may be straightforward, especially with infections of the femoral component, where swelling, heat, tenderness, a pulsatile mass, or possibly a draining sinus tract may be noted. However, the clinical presentation of an intracavitary graft infection may be non-specific and temporally remote (up to 10 years after surgery). Such non-specific presentations as malaise, back pain, and fever are usually absent. These patients are more likely to present with signs of complications of aortic graft infection, such as false aneurysm, gastrointestinal bleeding, elevated sedimentation rate, hydronephrosis, or ischaemia from a clotted graft. These should all be considered as potential manifestations of a graft infection and warrant further diagnostic evaluation. In early-onset infections, the patient may be systemically toxic with fever and leukocytosis. Bloodstream infection, wound infection, abdominal discomfort and graft dysfunction from recent thrombosis or anastomotic bleeding may also occur.[43]

MRSA has been increasingly implicated as a cause of postoperative wound infections, neurosurgical site infections and also endovascular prosthesis infection (such as cardiac stents, pacemakers, etc.) and no site is sacrosanct.

Conclusions

MRSA is an additional burden of infection to surgical and medical patients. It does not replace MSSA infection so arguments about whether it is more serious than MSSA infection are in many ways redundant. For the clinician, it remains a challenge for the foreseeable future and is likely to become even more pathogenic and antibiotic resistant.

References

1. Diekema DJ, Pfaller MA, Schmitz FJ et al.; and the SENTRY Participants Group. Survey of infections due to Staphylococcus species: frequency of occurrence and antimicrobial susceptibility of isolates collected in the United States, Canada, Latin America, Europe, and the Western Pacific region for the SENTRY Antimicrobial Surveillance Program, 1997–1999. Clin Infect Dis 2001; **32 (Suppl 2)**: S114-32.

2. Garner JS, Jarvis WR, Emori TG, Horan TC, Hughes JM. CDC definitions for nosocomial infections, 1988. Am J Infect Control 1988; **16**: 128–40.

3. Hoban DJ, Biedenbach DJ, Mutnick AH, Jones RN. Pathogen of occurrence and susceptibility patterns associated with pneumonia in hospitalized patients in North America: results of the SENTRY Antimicrobial Surveillance Study (2000). Diagn Microbiol Infect Dis 2003; **45**: 279–85.

4. Lowy FD. Staphylococcus aureus infections. N Engl J Med 1998; **339**: 520–32.

5. Noskin GA, Rubin RJ, Schentag JJ et al. The burden of Staphylococcus aureus infections on hospitals in the United States: an analysis of the 2000 and 2001 Nationwide Inpatient Sample Database. Arch Intern Med 2005; **165**: 1756–61.

6. Kuehnert MJ, Hill HA, Kupronis BA, Tokars JI, Solomon SL, Jernigan DB. Methicillin-resistant-*Staphylococcus aureus* hospitalizations, United States. *Emerg Infect Dis* 2005; **11**: 868–72.

7. Hershow RC, Khayr WF, Smith NL. A comparison of clinical virulence of nosocomially acquired methicillin-resistant and methicillin-sensitive *Staphylococcus aureus* infections in a university hospital. *Infect Control Hosp Epidemiol* 1992; **13**: 587–93.

8. Whitby M, McLaws M-L, Berry G. Risk of death from methicillin-resistant *Staphylococcus aureus* bacteraemia: a meta-analysis. *Med J Aust* 2001; **175**: 264–7.

9. Cosgrove SE, Sakoulas G, Perencevich EN, Schwaber MJ, Karchmer AW, Carmeli Y. Comparison of mortality associated with methicillin-resistant and methicillin-susceptible *Staphylococcus aureus* bacteremia: a meta-analysis. *Clin Infect Dis* 2003; **36**: 53–9.

10. Cheng, AF, French GL. Methicillin-resistant *Staphylococcus aureus* bacteraemia in Hong Kong. *J Hosp Infect* 1988; **12**: 91–101.

11. Mizushima Y, Kawasaki A, Hirata H *et al.* An analysis of bacteraemia in a university hospital in Japan over a 10-year period. *J Hosp Infect* 1994; **27**: 285–98.

12. Safdar N, Maki DG. The commonality of risk factors for nosocomial colonization and infection with antimicrobial-resistant *Staphylococcus aureus*, enterococcus, Gram-negative bacilli, *Clostridium difficile*, and *Candida*. *Ann Intern Med* 2002; **136**: 834–44.

13. Fishbain JT, Lee JC, Nguyen HD *et al.* Nosocomial transmission of methicillin-resistant *Staphylococcus aureus*: a blinded study to establish baseline acquisition rates. *Infect Control Hosp Epidemiol* 2003; **24**: 415–21.

14. Pujol M, Pena C, Pallares R *et al.* Nosocomial *Staphylococcus aureus* bacteremia among nasal carriers of methicillin-resistant and methicillin-susceptible strains. *Am J Med* 1996; **100**: 509–16.

15. Fridkin SK, Hageman JC, Morrison M *et al.* Methicillin-resistant *Staphylococcus aureus* disease in three communities. *N Engl J Med* 2005; **352**: 1436–44.

16. Wyllie DH, Peto TE, Crook D. MRSA bacteraemia in patients on arrival in hospital: a cohort study in Oxfordshire 1997–2003. *BMJ* 2005; **331**: 992.

17. Zetola N, Francis JS, Nuermberger EL, Bishai WR. Community-acquired meticillin-resistant *Staphylococcus aureus*: an emerging threat. *Lancet Infect Dis* 2005; **5**: 275–86.

18. Olson MM, Lee Jr JT. Continuous, 10-year wound infection surveillance. Results, advantages, and unanswered questions. *Arch Surg* 1990; **125**: 794–803.

19. Vincent JL, Bihari DJ, Suter PM *et al.* The prevalence of nosocomial infection in intensive care units in Europe. Results of the European Prevalence of Infection in Intensive Care (EPIC) Study. EPIC International Advisory Committee. *JAMA* 1995; **274**: 639–44.

20. Eggimann P, Pittet D. Overview of catheter-related infections with special emphasis on prevention based on educational programs. *Clin Microbiol Infect* 2002; **8**: 295–309.

21. Mermel LA, Farr BM, Sherertz RJ *et al.* Guidelines for the management of intravascular catheter-related infections. *Clin Infect Dis* 2001; **32**: 1249–72.

22. Francioli P, Masur H. Complications of *Staphylococcus aureus* bacteremia. Occurrence in patients undergoing long-term hemodialysis. *Arch Intern Med* 1982; **142**: 1655–8.

23. Harbarth S, Rutschmann O. Impact of methicillin resistance on the outcome of patients with bacteremia caused by *Staphylococcus aureus*. *Arch Intern Med* 1998; **158**: 182–9.

24. Cosgrove SE, Qi Y, Kaye KS, Harbarth S, Karchmer AW, Carmeli Y. The impact of methicillin resistance in *Staphylococcus aureus* bacteremia on patient outcomes: mortality, length of stay, and hospital charges. *Infect Control Hosp Epidemiol* 2005; **26**: 166–74.

25. Fowler Jr VG, Miro JM, Hoen B *et al. Staphylococcus aureus* endocarditis: a consequence of medical progress. *JAMA* 2005; **293**: 3012–21.

26. Lodise Jr TP, McKinnon PS, Rybak M. Prediction model to identify patients with *Staphylococcus aureus* bacteremia at risk for methicillin resistance. *Infect Control Hosp Epidemiol* 2003; **24**: 655–61.

27. Netzer ROM, Altwegg SC, Zollinger E, Täuber M, Carrel T, Seiler C. Infective endocarditis: determinants of long term outcome. *Heart* 2002; **88**: 61–6.

28. Fowler Jr VG, Sanders LL, Kong LK *et al.* Infective endocarditis due to *Staphylococcus aureus*: 59 prospectively identified cases with follow-up. *Clin Infect Dis* 1999; **28**: 106–14.

29. Nolan CM, Beaty HN. *Staphylococcus aureus* bacteremia. Current clinical patterns. *Am J Med* 1976; **60**: 495–500.

30. Bayer AS, Lam K, Ginzton L, Norman DC, Chiu CY, Ward JI. *Staphylococcus aureus* bacteremia. Clinical, serologic, and echocardiographic findings in patients with and without endocarditis. *Arch Intern Med* 1987; **147**: 457–62.

31. Chang CF, Kuo BI, Chen TL, Yang WC, Lee SD, Lin CC. Infective endocarditis in maintenance hemodialysis patients: fifteen years' experience in one medical center. *J Nephrol* 2004; **17**: 228–35.

32. Chang F-Y. *Staphylococcus aureus* bacteremia and endocarditis. *J Microbiol Immunol Infect* 2000; **33**: 63–8.

33. Chang F-Y, MacDonald BB, Peacock Jr JE *et al.* A prospective multicenter study of *Staphylococcus aureus* bacteremia: incidence of endocarditis, risk factors for mortality, and clinical impact of methicillin resistance. *Medicine (Baltimore)* 2003; **82**: 322–32.

34. Tak T, Reed KD, Haselby RC, McCauley Jr CS, Shukla SK. An update on the epidemiology, pathogenesis and management of infective endocarditis with emphasis on *Staphylococcus aureus*. *Wisconsin Med J* 2002; **101**: 24–33.

35. Dubost JJ, Soubrier M, De Champs C, Ristori JM, Bussiére JL, Sauvezie B. No changes in the distribution of organisms responsible for septic arthritis over a 20 year period. *Ann Rheum Dis* 2002; **61**: 267–9.

36. Gupta MN, Sturrock RD, Field M. Prospective comparative study of patients with culture proven and high suspicion of adult onset septic arthritis. *Ann Rheum Dis* 2003; **62**: 327–31.

37. Cleeman E, Auerbach JD, Klingenstein GG, Flatow EL. Septic arthritis of the glenohumeral joint: a review of 23 cases. *J Surg Orthop Adv* 2005; **14**: 102–7.

38. Priest DH, Peacock Jr JE. Hematogenous vertebral osteomyelitis due to *Staphylococcus aureus* in the adult: clinical features and therapeutic outcomes. *South Med J* 2005; **98**: 854–62.

39. Shams WE, Rapp RP. Methicillin-resistant staphylococcal infections: an important consideration for orthopedic surgeons. *Orthopedics* 2004; **27**: 565–8.

40. Jelic I, Anic D, Alfirevic I *et al*. Wound infection after median sternotomy during the war in Croatia. *J Cardiovasc Surg (Torino)* 1996; **37 (Suppl 1)**: 183–7.

41. Rello J, Sole-Violan J, Sa-Borges M *et al*. Pneumonia caused by oxacillin-resistant *Staphylococcus aureus* treated with glycopeptides. *Crit Care Med* 2005; **33**: 1983–7.

42. Naylor AR, Hayes PD, Darke S. A prospective audit of complex wound and graft infections in Great Britain and Ireland: the emergence of MRSA. *Eur J Vasc Endovasc Surg* 2001; **21**: 289–94.

43. FitzGerald SF, Kelly C, Humphreys H. Diagnosis and treatment of prosthetic aortic graft infections: confusion and inconsistency in the absence of evidence or consensus. *J Antimicrob Chemother* 2005; **56**: 996–9.

44. Naimi TS, LeDell KH, Como-Sabetti K *et al*. Comparison of community- and health care-associated methicillin-resistant *Staphylococcus aureus* infection. *JAMA* 2003; **290**: 2976–84.

45. Solomkin JS, Bjornson HS, Cainzos M *et al*. A consensus statement on empiric therapy for suspected Gram-positive infections in surgical patients. *Am J Surg* 2004; **187**: 134–45.

10. Treatment of MRSA infection

Ian M Gould, Abhijit M Bal

Antibiotics for treatment of MRSA infection
Practical considerations in the treatment of MRSA
Screening for MRSA carriage and decontamination

Staphylococci belong to the family Micrococcaceae and are divided into two broad categories of medical importance – *Staphylococcus aureus* that is coagulase positive and a group of staphylococci that give negative reaction with the coagulase test. This latter group of coagulase-negative staphylococci contains several species that cause infections in the immunocompromised host and those with prosthetic devices. *S. aureus* is a major cause of serious clinical infections that range from superficial infections of the integument to invasive and deep-organ involvement such as endocarditis and joint infections.

Soon after its discovery in 1941, penicillin was widely used in the treatment of staphylococcal and streptococcal infections. Resistance to penicillin, secondary to the production of the enzyme β-lactamase appeared soon thereafter. At present, almost all strains of *S. aureus* isolated from clinical specimens are resistant to penicillin. As a result of resistance to penicillin, a novel group of β-lactam antibiotics were developed that had low affinity to the β-lactamase enzyme. Consequently, these drugs were stable to the action of β-lactamases and included cloxacillin, dicloxacillin, flucloxacillin, methicillin, nafcillin and oxacillin. Wide-spread

and inappropriate use of some of these agents such as flucloxacillin and nafcillin led to selection of *S. aureus* mutants that had an altered structure of penicillin binding protein (PBP) thereby rendering them resistant to all penicillins and cephalosporins. PBPs are important enzymes that cross-link the peptidoglycan cell wall of Gram-positive bacteria. Genetic mutations in *S. aureus* lead to the acquisition of the *mecA* gene, which codes for PBP2a that has poor affinity to the β-lactam antibiotics. These organisms, on account of being methicillin resistant, are known as methicillin-resistant *S. aureus* or MRSA. MRSA is consequently resistant not only to methicillin but to all the available β-lactam antibiotics. As a result, once established, MRSA strains are further selected because of wide-spread use of broad-spectrum β-lactam antibiotics such as the third generation cephalosporins and quinolones. Because of the limited therapeutic options and a lack of response to the standard empiric regimens, MRSA is a serious problem in patients with clinical infections that need therapy. Uninfected but colonised individuals can easily transmit the organisms to those who are not colonised. In hospitalised patients, colonisation frequently leads to infection. There seems to be a much greater risk of infection in individuals colonised with MRSA than those colonised with methicillin-sensitive *S. aureus* (MSSA). In one study, 50% of MRSA carriers developed infection when followed up for 18 months and, in an intensive care setting, this could occur within a few days. Mortality rates are also much greater for infections caused by MRSA as compared to MSSA.

> MRSA is a serious problem in patients with clinical infections that need therapy. Uninfected, but colonised, individuals can easily transmit the organisms to those who are not colonised.

There seems to be a much greater risk of infection in individuals colonised with MRSA than those colonised with MSSA.

Antibiotics for treatment of MRSA infection

A semisynthetic penicillin such as flucloxacillin is generally the antibiotic of choice for the treatment of infections due to *S. aureus* that are sensitive to the β-lactamase stable penicillins. In serious infections due to MRSA, the glycopeptide antibiotics (vancomycin and teicoplanin) are the drugs most widely used though they are less active than flucloxacillin for strains that are sensitive to both drugs. Additionally, there are other agents that can be used either on their own (linezolid, quinupristin–dalfopristin, daptomycin) or along with the glycopeptides (rifampicin, gentamicin). However, none of the newer agents have clearly and consistently been shown to be better than glycopeptides. Moreover, deep-seated infections such as endocarditis are best treated with antibiotics known to have a bactericidal activity (Tables 10.1 and 10.2).

> Deep-seated infections such as endocarditis are best treated with antibiotics known to have a bactericidal activity.

The newer agents are likely to be useful for the expanding number of infections caused by MRSA that have a higher minimum inhibitory concentration (MIC) to glycopeptides (glycopeptide-intermediate *S. aureus* [GISA] or vancomycin-resistant *S. aureus* [VRSA]). Strains of the latter type have not been isolated in the UK.

Glycopeptides and related compounds

Vancomycin is the treatment of choice for serious MRSA infections. Vancomycin binds to D-alanine, a component of the peptidoglycan in the Gram-positive bacterial cell wall. Binding of vancomycin to this molecule leads to the inhibition of cell wall synthesis and bacterial death. However, vancomycin is weakly

Table 10.1
Antibiotics for MRSA

Glycopeptides	Older agents that are frequently active
Vancomycin	Gentamicin
Teicoplanin	Tetracyclines
Dalbavancin	Fusidic acid
Oritavancin	Cotrimoxazole
Telavancin	Rifampicin*
Ramoplanin	
Oxazolidinones	Topical antimicrobial agents
Linezolid	Mupirocin*
Ranbezolid	Tyrothricin
	Bacitracin
	Gramicidin
	Chlorhexidine**
	Povidone iodine**
	Hydrogen peroxide**
Streptogramins	
Quinupristin–dalfopristin	
Lipopeptides	
Daptomycin	
Glycylcyclines	
Tigecycline	

Agents in development are italicised.
*Resistance can be a problem; **antiseptic.

bactericidal as compared to flucloxacillin. Teicoplanin is also widely used for the treatment of MRSA infections. As compared to vancomycin, teicoplanin has a longer half-life but also has a higher protein binding thus decreasing the number of free molecules available to act on the bacterial cells. Also, while assays for measuring vancomycin trough levels are widely available, this is not the case with teicoplanin. Consequently, less information is available regarding dosages and the safety profile for teicoplanin; this often leads to the use of a sub-therapeutic dosing for serious infections. There are several drawbacks to therapy with glycopeptides. Glycopeptide monotherapy is often inadequate in serious clinical infections and addition of other agents such as rifampicin is usually recommended for MRSA endocarditis and pneumonia. Vancomycin is potentially both nephrotoxic and ototoxic and levels need to be monitored. Trough levels can be used as a guide to both toxicity and efficacy. Also, both drugs are available only as parenteral agents (oral vancomycin, available for treatment of antibiotic-associated colitis is not absorbed) that in practice limit the options for therapy outwith the hospital.

> Vancomycin is the antibiotic of choice for serious MRSA infections but glycopeptide monotherapy is often inadequate in serious infections and addition of agents such as rifampicin is recommended for MRSA endocarditis and pneumonia.

Due to the lack of alternative agents of proven value, glycopeptides are likely to remain the mainstay of therapy for MRSA infections for some time. Newer glycopeptides in development include oritavancin, telavancin and dalbavancin. Dalbavancin has a long half-life and once weekly administration is probably adequate. However, potential disadvantages of a long half-life include development of resistance over the period of time during which the drug may have levels lower than its MIC, and also the management of anaphylactic reactions. Long-acting glycopeptides could prove very useful as part of an out-patient,

home-based antibiotic therapy, thus decreasing the duration of stay in the hospital. A related compound, a lipoglycodepsipeptide called ramoplanin, also inhibits peptidoglycan synthesis. Ramoplanin binds to the lipid intermediates in the peptidoglycan chain thus inhibiting the late stages in peptidoglycan synthesis. It is rapidly bactericidal for MRSA.

> Less information is available regarding dosage and the safety profile for teicoplanin; this often leads to the use of a sub-therapeutic dosing for serious infections.

Oxazolidinones

Linezolid is the most important new agent that has so far been introduced for the treatment of MRSA infections. It belongs to the oxazolidinone group of antibiotics and was licensed in January 2001 in the UK. It is bacteriostatic for S. aureus and acts by binding to the 50S ribosomal subunit thereby preventing the synthesis of the 70S subunit. The drug can be administered both orally and intravenously. Its major advantages are excellent tissue penetration and its oral absorption that approaches 100%. The drug should be used with caution in patients with abnormal liver function tests. Thrombocytopenia is a major adverse effect of linezolid. Marrow toxicity is more common in elderly patients, in diabetics, in alcoholics and in those with pre-treatment haemoglobin of less than 10.5 g/dl. There is some evidence that linezolid is better than vancomycin for the empirical treatment of nosocomial pneumonia. Combined data of two trials showed a better survival rate in the subset of patients found to have MRSA pneumonia who were on linezolid than in those who were on vancomycin. However, data derived from subset analysis should be interpreted with caution, as the subsets could not be randomised. Also, each of the two individual prospective studies that were combined to obtain these retrospective data did not show any benefit. Linezolid has also been found to be superior to teicoplanin in the treatment of Gram-positive bacterial infections and the difference was most notable for bacteraemic infections. Teicoplanin was used at a dose of 400 mg/day and, as discussed above, a higher dose could possibly have led to a different outcome. Patients on teicoplanin had fewer side-effects than those on linezolid. Linezolid has also been used for the treatment of prosthetic joint infections caused by MRSA. Joint infections usually need prolonged treatment, often up to 6 weeks, even in situations where two-stage revision operations are planned. The toxicity of linezolid could be higher in patients treated for longer than 4 weeks and the manufacturer does not recommend therapy for longer than 4 weeks. Reversible peripheral neuropathy and optic neuritis have been documented with prolonged treatment. If a decision to use linezolid is made, baseline haematological values should be obtained and regular monitoring should be undertaken. Linezolid is an available option for the treatment of GISA infections. Linezolid has been successfully used with aminoglycosides, such as amikacin, in the treatment of GISA endocarditis although there is paucity of data to support such combinations and the drug is only bacteriostatic. Reports of linezolid resistance in both *S. aureus* and *E. faecium* have already appeared in the literature and this is probably more likely with prolonged therapy. Unfortunately, conditions such as endocarditis, osteomyelitis and prosthetic joint infections need to be treated for at least 6 weeks. When such prolonged therapy is required, linezolid should be used only when safer options are not available. It is useful to have a clear local guideline on use of this agent and expert microbiology advice should always be sought.

> There is some evidence that linezolid is better than vancomycin for the empirical treatment of nosocomial pneumonia.

Streptogramins

Quinupristin–dalfopristin belongs to the streptogramin group of antibiotics. The drug is

bactericidal. Resistance to the quinupristin component makes the agent bacteriostatic while resistance to dalfopristin components makes the entire molecule ineffective. Resistance can occur secondary to ribosomal target modification (quinupristin), enzyme inactivation (both quinupristin and dalfopristin) or an efflux mechanism (dalfopristin). Ribosomal target modification is commonly manifested as macrolide-lincosamide-streptogramin B (MLSB) phenotype encoded by the *erm* genes; this makes the strains resistant not only to quinupristin but also the macrolides (erythromycin) and lincosamides (clindamycin). Quinupristin–dalfopristin is available only for intravenous administration. In murine models of MRSA and GISA pneumonia, quinupristin–dalfopristin has been shown to be superior to vancomycin. In a study on patients in intensive care who had previously failed vancomycin therapy, quinupristin–dalfopristin was shown to be effective but several studies suggest a high rate of phlebitis. However, data are insufficient to recommend a role for quinupristin–dalfopristin in the treatment of MRSA infections. It can be used in selective cases of GISA infections if the patients are intolerant to linezolid. Quinupristin–dalfopristin is available only as an intravenous agent. A related compound, pristinamycin, is available for oral use in France where it has been used with some success.

> There is insufficient data to recommend a role for quinupristin–dalfopristin in the treatment of MRSA infection.

Lipopeptides

> Daptomycin has recently been licensed in the UK for the treatment of skin and soft-tissue infection with *S. aureus*.

Daptomycin belongs to another new class of agents recently licensed in the UK for the treatment of skin and soft-tissue infection with

S. aureus. It has an excellent bactericidal activity for Gram-positive bacteria that may lead to shorter treatment courses. It acts by depleting the cell membrane potential without lysing the membrane itself. Daptomycin resistant isolates have been obtained from patients on prolonged daptomycin therapy. The drug is also contra-indicated for the treatment of pneumonia as it interacts with pulmonary surfactant. Its use remains to be defined at the present time but it is hoped it will also prove successful in bacteraemia and deep-seated infection such as endocarditis and osteomyelitis. Daptomycin is administered once daily and this makes it a useful agent for out-patient-based treatment. Reversible myopathy of the skeletal muscles is an important adverse effect of daptomycin therapy. Creatine phosphokinase (CPK) levels need to be monitored during therapy.

Glycylcyclines

Tigecycline is a glycylcycline antibiotic that binds to the 30S ribosome of both Gram-positive and Gram-negative bacteria. Unlike other new agents developed for MRSA, tigecycline has a broad spectrum of activity excluding *Pseudomonas* spp. It is bacteriostatic. In a phase III trial, it was found to have an activity similar to vancomycin plus aztreonam for skin and soft-tissue infections. It is now available for treatment of skin, soft-tissue and intra-abdominal infections. Tigecycline is potentially useful in intensive care settings as an empirical choice for infections that include MRSA. It has a very good tissue penetration but is rapidly cleared from blood. It remains to be established whether this pharmacokinetic profile will limit its use in patients with septicaemia.

> Tigecycline has a broad spectrum of activity unlike other new agents developed for MRSA.

Other agents in development

A number of promising agents that are active against MRSA are on the horizon. MRSA is resistant to β-lactams on account of mutation in PBP2. The mutated PBP2 called, PBP2a has lower affinity to the β-lactam group of antibiotics. In theory, it should be possible to generate synthetic β-lactams that bind to the altered form of PBP2. Ceftobiprole is a new cephalosporin that is now entering phase III trials. It has a high affinity to PBP2a. It is also active against vancomycin intermediate strains of MRSA and, like tigecycline, has a broad spectrum of activity. Newer oxazolidinones such as ranbezolid, useful against staphylococci, are effective in penetrating biofilms. A new dihydrofolate reductase inhibitor, iclaprim, may also be available in the future. It has been found to retain activity against staphylococci that are resistant to trimethoprim. Another group of compounds called stemphones have been found to enhance the potency of carbapenems such as imipenem against MRSA (Table 10.2).

Practical considerations in the treatment of MRSA

An important question that frequently arises is when to treat patients with MRSA. If a patient has MRSA isolated with symptoms of infection, they are said to be infected. In the absence of symptoms, they are said to be colonised.

Table 10.2
Properties of antibiotics for MRSA

Bactericidal agents
- Daptomycin
- Quinupristin–dalfopristin
- Rifampicin*
- Ceftobiprole

Weakly bactericidal agents
- Vancomycin
- Teicoplanin

Bacteriostatic
- Linezolid
- Tigecycline*
- Trimethoprim
- Fusidic acid
- Tetracyclines

*Good activity in biofilms.

Invasive infections including bloodstream infections, deep-organ infections and infections of prosthetic devices should always be treated urgently, preferably with bactericidal antibiotics.

Most such infections require combination treatment to eradicate the MRSA while preventing emergence of resistant clones. Often, treatment needs to be prolonged with thorough debridement and removal of prosthesis. The laboratory must make sure that all appropriate antibiotics are tested for the MRSA strain. It may be prudent to preserve such strains for typing so that the mechanism of spread can be understood and appropriate control measures instituted. Also, additional susceptibility tests at a later date may become necessary.

In most circumstances, isolation of MRSA from cultures taken through intravascular devices is an indication for line removal. A brief course of vancomycin following removal of such devices is commonly administered though its value has never been established. Similarly, removal of drains at an appropriate time may lead to eradication of MRSA from local sites. It is noteworthy that MRSA wound infections commonly seen at out-patient units in surgical practice can usually be treated with oral and cost-effective antibiotics, such as trimethoprim, fusidic acid or doxycycline, subject to local susceptibility pattern. A combination of two oral agents is usually recommended to prevent further emergence of resistance. Unfortunately, costly oral agents such as linezolid are often inappropriately used in these circumstances and such wide-spread and irrational use can only generate resistance making it impossible to treat serious infections where the newer drugs are needed. MRSA infection of the urinary tract can be treated with oral nitrofurantoin or a tetracycline in the absence of a catheter although susceptibility needs to be confirmed. Trimethoprim–sulphamethoxazole combination is probably satisfactory for moderately severe MRSA infections if the strain is susceptible to each of the two components.

Serious infections such as endocarditis and osteomyelitis are best treated with a combination of two agents for a prolonged period. The treatment of central nervous system infections such as brain abscess is particularly challenging, as the penetration of vancomycin in the cerebrospinal fluid is uncertain. Combination treatment with vancomycin and rifampicin is indicated for such infections. In meningitis associated with ventriculo-peritoneal shunt, intraventricular administration of vancomycin following externalisation via a ventricular drainage is recommended to compensate for the uncertain penetration of systemic vancomycin. In the emerging community acquired MRSA infections, clinical presentation can vary from mild furunculosis that requires only an incision and drainage to severe necrotising fasciitis or pneumonia where antibiotics such as linezolid or clindamycin (provided the strain is susceptible) which are thought to reduce toxin production may be the best drugs.

Screening for MRSA carriage and decontamination

In the absence of clear signs of infections, patients are said to be colonised but they are often treated in the hope that eradication of MRSA would be achieved. In the presence of open wound drains, central lines and long-term venous access devices that need to be preserved, successful eradication will probably never be achieved. Patients infected and subsequently treated for MRSA should be screened for MRSA carriage in the anterior nares and other sites such as perineum, axilla and throat. Attempts at eradication guided by these results will often be successful. Such a 'seek and destroy' policy (see chapter by Seaton) may help prevent the spread of MRSA strains both in the hospital and in the community and decrease the overall burden of MRSA carriage. Infection control procedures in the hospital prevent the intrahospital spread of the organism from index cases to other patients and help reduce the burden of infection, reduce the length of hospital stay and decrease cost. Unfortunately, the compliance rate for measures such as hand washing and barrier nursing is poor and in specific settings of high risk, such as intensive care units, temporary patient decontamination with antiseptics can reduce the hazard that such patients pose to others.

Further reading

Fowler VG, Boucher HW, Corey G et al. Daptomycin versus standard therapy for bacteraemia and endocarditis caused by *Staphylococcus aureus*. *N Engl J Med* 2006; **355**: 653–65.

Gemmell CG, Edwards DI, Fraise AP et al. Guidelines for the prophylaxis and treatment of methicillin-resistant *Staphylococcus aureus* (MRSA) infections in the UK. *J Antimicrob Chemother* 2006; **57**: 589–608.

Gould IM. Control of methicillin-resistant *Staphylococcus aureus* in the UK. *Eur J Clin Microbiol Infect Dis* 2005; **24**: 789–93.

Gould IM. The clinical significance of methicillin-resistant *Staphylococcus aureus*. *J Hosp Infect* 2005; **61**: 277–82.

Gould IM. The costs of MRSA and its control. *Int J Antimicrob Agents* 2006; In Press.

Livermore DM. Can beta-lactams be re-engineered to beat MRSA? *Clin Microbiol Infect* 2006; **12 (Suppl 2)**: 11–6.

Moreillon P, Al Que Y, Glauser MP. *Staphylococcus aureus* (including staphylococcal toxic shock syndrome). In: Mandell GL, Bennett JE, Dolin R. (eds) *Mandell, Douglas and Bennett's Principles and Practice of Infectious Diseases*, 6th edn. Philadelphia, PA: Elsevier Churchill Livingstone, 2005; 2321–51.

Rybak MJ. The efficacy and safety of daptomycin: first in a new class of antibiotics for Gram-positive bacteria. *Clin Microbiol Infect* 2006; **12 (Suppl 1)**: 24–32.

Wilcox M, Nathwani D, Dryden M. Linezolid compared with teicoplanin for the treatment of suspected or proven Gram-positive infections. *J Antimicrob Chemother* 2004; **53**: 335–44.

Wilcox MH. Tigecycline and the need for a new broad-spectrum antibiotic class. *Surg Infect (Larchmt)* 2006; **7**: 69–80.

Wilcox MH. Update on linezolid: the first oxazolidinone antibiotic. *Expert Opin Pharmacother* 2005; **6**: 2315–26.

Wunderink RG, Rello J, Cammarata SK et al. Linezolid vs vancomycin: analysis of two double-blind studies of patients with methicillin-resistant *Staphylococcus aureus* nosocomial pneumonia. *Chest* 2003; **124**: 1789–97.

11. Decolonisation of MRSA patients

R Andrew Seaton

The consequences of MRSA colonisation

Agents used to decolonise patients with MRSA

Is it possible to eradicate MRSA colonisation?

Is it possible to prevent MRSA infection through decolonisation strategies?

How should MRSA-colonised patients be managed?

Colonisation with *Staphylococcus aureus* refers to transient or persistent, asymptomatic bacterial carriage which is not implicated in an acute or chronic infection. Sites normally associated with colonisation are non-sterile and include the anterior nares, wounds, skin ulcers, axillae, throat and perineum. It is important to differentiate carriage from infection which could be defined as the isolation of *S. aureus* from an inflamed site or a normally sterile site (*e.g.* joint space or blood). Rates of colonisation vary greatly but about 30% of hospitalised adults may be colonised with *S. aureus* at any time. The proportion of patients colonised with methicillin-resistant *S. aureus* (MRSA) will depend on the nature and diversity of the hospital population as well as the local implementation of infection control measures. Rates of MRSA bacteraemia, which are usually recorded by hospitals, tend to correlate with colonisation rates. In outbreak situations, MRSA colonisation rates may change rapidly and may exceed the normal *S aureus* carriage rate, particularly in extranasal sites. Many factors may affect MRSA colonisation. Higher rates are associated with units where patient turnover is greatest, invasive procedures are most prevalent, where patients with renal disease and diabetes are concentrated and antibiotic consumption, particularly of the cephalosporins and fluoroquinolones, is greatest (Table 11.1). Staffing levels and patient movement/boarding are also likely to be important factors affecting MRSA colonisation rates. Clearly, where hand disinfection prior to and following patient contact is poor, MRSA rates are higher. Improved availability of alcohol-based gel for hand disinfection is associated with lower rates of MRSA colonisation and also healthcare-associated infection. Inadequate cleaning of near patient sites such as 'cot-sides', radiators, door handles, *etc.* may be associated with increased carriage rates. Near-site contamination also increases the risk of re-colonisation following MRSA eradication.

Colonisation refers to transient or persistent, asymptomatic bacterial carriage at a non-sterile and uninflamed site.

The consequences of MRSA colonisation

Up to one in three of MRSA-colonised patients will subsequently require treatment for an MRSA infection.

Table 11.1
Patient factors associated with MRSA colonisation

- Prior colonisation/infection with MRSA
- Diabetes mellitus
- Renal dialysis
- (Cardio)vascular disease
- Recent or prolonged antibiotic therapy (particularly with fluoroquinolones and cephalosporins)
- Prolonged or recurrent hospital admission
- Nursing home resident
- Admission to intensive care or high dependency unit
- Central venous catheter *in situ*

By definition colonisation does no immediate harm to patients. However, up to one in three of such patients will subsequently require treatment for an MRSA infection (Fig. 11.1) either in relation to the site of the colonisation (*e.g.* wound infection) or at a distant sites (*e.g.* prosthetic joint infection). Patients in hospitals may be particularly vulnerable to infection by *S. aureus* (including MRSA); once colonised, infection may follow through skin breaches, vascular access devices, urinary catheters, nasogastric feeding tubes and endotracheal tubes. Risk of MRSA infection in the colonised patient, therefore, is related to a patient's dependency and clinical status, *i.e.* elderly or immune-compromised patients in high dependency or intensive care or undergoing dialysis are at greatest risk. Citing of central venous catheters is an independent risk factor for bacteraemia in those colonised. In the intensive care setting, MRSA colonisation has been observed to pose a 4-fold increased risk of bacteraemia compared to the risk in those colonised with methicillin-sensitive *Staphylococcus aureus* (MSSA). In view of the infection risk following colonisation, it is important that all colonised patients are assessed for signs of infection. Likewise, if symptoms of infection arise in an MRSA colonised patient, MRSA should be considered in the aetiology of the clinical syndrome.

> Central venous catheters are an independent risk factor for bacteraemia in those colonised with MRSA.

If symptoms of infection arise in an MRSA-colonised patient, MRSA should be considered in the aetiology of the clinical syndrome.

As well as being at risk of MRSA infection, those colonised serve as an 'MRSA reservoir' for healthcare workers and patients. Onwards transmission of MRSA may occur via direct contact with healthcare workers, via contamination of the environment or via aerosol.

Agents used to decolonise patients with MRSA

Eradication of MRSA from the hospitalised patient clearly would be advantageous – both to the patient and to the hospital environment. Decolonisation therapy usually consists of a topical antibacterial applied carefully to the anterior nares twice or thrice daily for 5–7 days, combined with an antiseptic body wash/shampoo applied daily. This regimen is combined with near-patient environmental cleaning and daily bedding, night wear and towel changes. The most frequently used and studied regimen consists of nasal mupirocin and chlorhexidene body wash. Side-effects are unusual and consist mainly of localised skin irritation. More severe side-effects are very rarely reported. Other topical agents have been evaluated such as nasal fucidin or tea-tree oil and triclosan or povodine-iodine body wash. Throat colonisation, which may be a reason for persistent nasal carriage, may occasionally be treated with chlorhexidene throat spray or throat 'gargle' but only on the advice of a specialist. Persistent carriage is a difficult clinical problem, particularly when it affects staff, and requires specialist management guided by a clinical microbiologist or infectious disease physician in conjunction with a

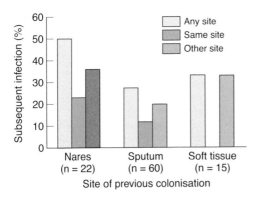

Figure 11.1
MRSA colonisation and risk of subsequent infection (adapted from Huang *et al.*, 2003).

specialist in occupational health (in the case of healthcare workers). Often, systemic therapy with two oral agents active against MRSA (*e.g.* rifampicin plus fucidin or trimethoprim or doxycycline or cotrimoxazole) is needed. In persistent carriers, gastrointestinal carriage should be considered, and this occasionally will require treatment with oral vancomycin, usually in combination with systemic therapy.

> Improved availability of alcohol-based gel for hand disinfection is associated with lower rates of MRSA colonisation and healthcare-associated infection.

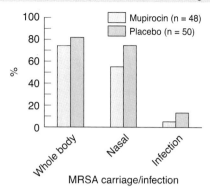

Figure 11.2
Effect of decolonisation therapy on MRSA carriage (adapted from Harbarth *et al.*, 1999).

When decolonisation strategies are used, they should be used in conjunction with other infection control measures including patient isolation, barrier nursing, hand disinfection and environmental cleaning.

Is it possible to eradicate MRSA colonisation?

No study has been performed, to date, which can robustly assess the efficacy of decolonisation therapy on patients with MRSA carriage. When decolonisation strategies are used, they should be used in conjunction with other infection control measures including patient isolation, barrier nursing, hand disinfection and environmental cleaning. In MRSA-colonised patients, chlorhexidene body wash combined with topical nasal mupirocin has been associated with eradication from the anterior nares in 44% compared to 23% receiving chlorhexidene body wash and placebo. Results from extra-nasal sites have been even less convincing (Fig. 11.2). Re-treatment of persistent carriers has been found to be largely unsuccessful and may be associated with the emergence of strains resistant to mupiricin. Any attempt at decolonisation should include removal or replacement of potentially colonised in-dwelling devices such as urinary catheters and vascular devices.

Although there is a lack of data on the long-term impact of MRSA decolonisation, a number of well-designed studies have been performed which show that a combination of chlorhexidene body wash and nasal mupiricin are superior to placebo in the short-term eradication of methicillin-sensitive *S. aureus*. About 85% of mupiricin recipients compared to 26% of placebo recipients are cleared of carriage after a single course of eradication therapy. In healthcare workers, nasal carriage of *S. aureus* has apparently been eliminated in nearly 90% of subjects with 5 days of therapy, compared to 10% with placebo. However re-colonisation has been observed at the rate of 43% at 1 month, 56% at 3 months and 67% at 6 months.

Is it possible to prevent MRSA infection through decolonisation strategies?

The only randomised, controlled study of decolonisation of MRSA was not powered to assess the impact on infection rates; therefore, no firm conclusions can be drawn (Fig. 11.2). Likewise, non-randomised, observational studies have not suggested reductions in infection rate with MRSA. Decolonisation strategies in general surgical and orthopaedic patients colonised with MSSA failed to show an overall significant reduction in clinically important surgical site infections although proven *S. aureus* infections may occur less frequently. In non-surgical patients colonised with *S. aureus*, decolonisation strategies have had no effect on the rate of subsequent infections, including proven *S. aureus* infections. The only group where there is some evidence of benefit of decolonisation is in patients receiving either peritoneal or haemodialysis, where topical mupiricin has been shown to reduce the incidence of staphylococcal infections.

> Large, randomised, controlled studies are required to evaluate the benefits of decolonisation therapy on patients colonised with MRSA.

How should MRSA-colonised patients be managed?

Policies should reflect local MRSA endemicity and potential cost-effectiveness. Hospitals with a low rate of MRSA carriage would be sensible to manage each new case as aggressively as possible – a so-called 'seek and destroy' policy. In hospitals where MRSA is endemic, the best management is less clear and is much debated. In these circumstances, it is not possible to make a robust, evidence-based argument for or against the routine decolonisation of patients with MRSA carriage. Although most MRSA infections are acquired from endogenous strains there will always be a risk of exogenous strains re-colonising or causing infection directly in the previously colonised patient who remains in hospital. It is essential, therefore, that decolonisation strategies are never considered alone and should always be employed in the context of a comprehensive infection control policy, which includes hand disinfection and isolation. At present, there are no clear data to justify routine eradication of MRSA in patients outside hospital including those in long-term care facilities.

Since the risk of MRSA infection is increased in colonised patients in hospital, and because of

the potential consequences of such infections, it does seem prudent to attempt to decolonise vulnerable hospitalised patients. Patients who may merit particular targeting, in view of the risk of deep-seated or surgical site infections, are those scheduled for joint replacement or (cardio)vascular surgery. Decolonisation in such patients ideally should be completed prior to hospital admission and they should be isolated in hospital on admission whenever possible. Patients with other risk factors for MRSA infection, such as those in high dependency or intensive care, would certainly benefit from eradication of MRSA. However, they are probably the least likely to respond to decolonisation treatment due to multisite involvement and the most likely to be re-colonised following treatment. Decolonisation therapy may offer short-term protection to patients at least some of the time although extra-nasal site colonisation is less likely to respond to treatment and relapse rates are high where in-dwelling devices are not removed.

> Patients with extra-nasal site colonisation with MRSA are unlikely to respond to topical decolonisation therapy.

Any attempt at decolonisation should include removal or replacement of potentially colonised in-dwelling devices such as urinary catheters and vascular devices.

The effect of MRSA decolonisation on reducing the risk of onward transmission to healthcare workers and other patients has not been studied in isolation from other infection control measures. For the time being, therefore, it should be included as an important infection control measure in outbreak situations. Management of the selected colonised patient is summarised in Table 11.2. In colonised patients undergoing surgery, as well as decolonisation therapy, peri-operative prophylactic antibiotic therapy (where indicated) should include an agent to cover MRSA (*e.g.* gentamicin or vancomycin).

Table 11.2
Management of the MRSA-colonised patient

- Perform a full MRSA screen (nares, wounds, ulcers, axillae, perineum [groin], throat)
- Assess and be vigilant for clinical signs of MRSA infection
- Remove or replace in-dwelling devices including central venous catheters whenever possible
- Isolate or cohort depending on patient numbers
- Nasal mupiricin twice or thrice daily for 5–7 days
- Chlorhexidene skin cleaning daily for 5–7 days
- Environmental cleaning and bedding/clothes changing daily
- Repeat screening after decolonisation therapy
- Peri-operative antibiotic prophylaxis against MRSA (*e.g.* intravenous vancomycin)

Further reading

Fernandez C, Gaspar C, Torrellas A et al. A double-blind placebo controlled clinical trial to evaluate the safety and efficacy of mupiricin calcium ointment for eliminating nasal carriage of Staphylococcus aureus among hospital personnel. *J Hosp Infect* 1995; **35**: 399–408.

Harbarth S, Dharan S, Liassine N, Herrault P, Aukenthaler R, Pittet D. Randomized, placebo-controlled, double-blind trial to evaluate the efficacy of mupiricin for eradicating carriage of methicillin-resistant *Staphylococcus aureus*. *Antimicrob Agents Chemother* 1999; **43**: 1412–6.

Huang SS, Platt R. Risk of MRSA infection after previous infection or colonisation. *Clin Infect Dis* 2003; **36**: 281–5.

Laupland KB, Conly JM. Treatment of *Staphylococcus aureus* colonization and prophylaxis for infection with topical intranasal mupiricin: an evidence-based review. *Clin Infect Dis* 2003; **37**: 933–8.

Perl TM, Cullen JJ, Wenzel RP et al. Intranasal mupiricin to prevent postoperative *Staphylococcus aureus* infections. *N Engl J Med* 2003; **346**: 1871–7.

Pujol M, Pena C, Pellares R et al. Nosocomial *Staphylococcus aureus* bacteremia among nasal carriage of methicillin-resistant and methicillin-sensitive strains. *Am J Med* 1996; **100**: 509–16.

Tacconelli E, Carmeli Y, Aizer A, Ferreira G, Foreman MG, D'Agata EMC. Mupiricin prophylaxis to prevent *Staphylococcus aureus* infection in patients undergoing dialysis: a meta-analysis. *Clin Infect Dis* 2003; **37**: 1629–38.

12. Alternative treatments for MRSA

Thomas V Riley

Medicinal plants

Essential oils

Honey

Bacteriophages as antimicrobial agents

Bacterial interference

Conclusions

With the emergence of antibiotic resistance as a major public health problem, and the apparent decline in pharmaceutical company drive to produce new antimicrobials, there has been an increase in interest in revisiting remedies and agents once popular before the advent of the antibiotic era.

This makes sense; it is obvious that many of these therapies worked hundreds if not thousands of years ago, although the scientific basis of some is rather obscure. With others, however, good data exist on both *in vitro* and *in vivo* efficacy. A few randomised clinical trials have been completed with good outcomes. There are several treatment modalities used in traditional medicine in which there has been major interest in the last 20 years to the extent that one, artesunate, has become an accepted therapy. Others include garlic, other plant extracts, essential oils, honey, bacteriophage therapy and bacterial interference. Two factors have been instrumental in driving this examination of alternative therapies. First is the ever-increasing problem of antibiotic resistance, and the related issue of pharmaceutical companies down-sizing anti-infective drug

development. More recently, however, the threat of bioterrorism has prompted governments, although mainly defence departments, to get involved in developing new strategies for the treatment of biothreats.

Since the early 1980s, microbiologists, infectious-disease physicians and infection-control practitioners in hospitals in many parts of the world have been pre-occupied with ever-increasing numbers of methicillin-resistant *Staphylococcus aureus* (MRSA). The recent appearance of decreased vancomycin susceptibility in strains of multiresistant MRSA, and then true resistance, caused great concern world-wide. Multiresistance has been common among MRSA until recently when strains of apparent community origin emerged in various parts of the world that were non-multiresistant. These strains appear to have been acquired prior to hospital admission, and with no other risk factors for MRSA acquisition. They have been reported predominantly in various groups of indigenous peoples, like Canadian Inuits and Australian Aboriginals, and in situations where there is close contact between individuals, such as in jails, military barracks, schools and sporting teams.

There is ample evidence that the increased use of antibiotics leads to greater antibiotic resistance. *S. aureus* is the most common cause of hospital-acquired infections and the potential for untreatable multiresistant MRSA infections is real.

Although some new antimicrobials have been developed progress is slow, and the early promise of immunotherapy of infectious diseases has not been fulfilled. This chapter describes several alternative approaches to conventional antibiotics for the treatment and prevention of infection, particularly infection with MRSA. While some of these approaches are quite experimental, and many are suitable only for topical therapy, others do offer a real alternative to conventional antimicrobials in certain situations, either as sole or adjunctive therapy

Medicinal plants

> Phytomedicines (plant-based remedies in the form of teas, extracts and oils) are a multimillion dollar industry world-wide, and many are targeted towards infectious diseases.

The antimicrobial activity of plant oils and extracts has formed the basis of many applications, including raw and processed food preservation, pharmaceuticals, alternative medicine and natural therapies. Over 2700 plant species are reported to be active against *S. aureus*, and many have specific activity against MRSA. A 50% ethanol extract of the dried fruits of *Terminalia chebula* inhibited the growth of MRSA with a minimum inhibitory concentration (MIC) of 31.3 µg/ml. This plant is found in South-East Asia and has been used traditionally to treat upper respiratory tract infections. The main constituents of the fruit are hydrolysable tannins. Berberine is a naturally occurring isoquinolone alkaloid present in a number of plants such as *Coptis chinensis* and *Berberis vulgaris*. Berberine will inhibit the growth of *S. aureus* with an MIC of 25 µg/ml. Various extracts of *Hypericum perforatum*, commonly known as St John's Wort, are also active against MRSA. Historically, St John's Wort has been used to treat skin and wound infections and the active component appears to be hyperforin, a phloroglucin. These are just a few examples of the many plants that have antimicrobial activity. Some of these plants have been in use for thousands of years and would appear safe; however, a lot more work is required on safety, particularly in relation to interactions with conventional medication.

Essential oils

Various publications have documented the antimicrobial activity of essential oils including rosewood, rosemary, peppermint, bay, basil, tea-tree, celery seed and fennel. Oils such as pumpkin, evening primrose, sweet almond, carrot and mandarin have little or no activity. This is not surprising as most of this latter group are fixed oils, which are largely used as diluents for essential oils or as sources of dietary fatty acids. A major problem with all essential oil antimicrobial work is that all recognised testing methodologies are designed for testing water-soluble compounds and oils do not fit into this category. Various methods have been used to accommodate oils in laboratory testing; however, the most popular is to introduce a small amount of surfactant to help with solubilising the oil. With appropriate controls this works well although too much surfactant can inhibit oil activity. Because of these methodological issues, together with the problem of oil quality, it is sometimes difficult to compare results from studies and caution is required when interpreting some findings.

> When investigations are carried out correctly, many plant essential oils have marked *in vitro* antistaphylococcal activity at low concentrations.

For example, the MICs for lemongrass, sandalwood, thyme and vetiver against *S. aureus* are 0.06% (v/v), 0.03%, 0.03% and 0.008%, respectively. Interestingly, sandalwood oil has a specific anti-Gram-positive effect with all Gram-negative bacteria tested having high MICs (> 8.0% v/v). In many ways, sandalwood oil behaves like New Zealand manuka oil (from *Leptospermum scoparium* and often referred to as New Zealand tea-tree oil) which also has marginal activity against Gram-negative organisms. Kanuka oil is extracted from another New Zealand plant, *Kunzea ericoides*, but has poor antimicrobial activity. The antimicrobial activity of essential oils is related to their composition. These oils comprise mainly monoterpenes, sesquiterpenes and related alcohols. The distillation process can markedly effect the final composition of the oils and few regulatory controls are in place world-wide to ensure quality.

Tea-tree oil

Most essential oil work has been done with Australian tea-tree oil, the essential oil extracted by steam distillation from an Australian native tree *Melaleuca alternifolia*. There is now a large and growing body of both laboratory and clinical data pertaining to its efficacy. A recent report in the *Medical Journal of Australia* stated: 'The experimental evidence supporting the use of tea tree oil as a prophylactic for MRSA is compelling'. As with many plant extracts, tea-tree oil is a complicated mixture of approximately 100 components, several of which have antimicrobial activity. Although the development of microbial resistance to tea-tree oil has been suggested, this is unlikely to occur because resistance to several components would have to occur simultaneously. Tea-tree oil has good *in vitro* activity against methicillin-susceptible and methicillin-resistant *S. aureus*.

Until recently, what had been lacking is any clinical trials data; however, this is changing. In a pilot study, a tea-tree oil nasal ointment/body wash combination was better than mupirocin/Triclosan for the eradication of MRSA carriage. Although the number of patients studied was small, and the differences were not statistically significant, the results were encouraging. A recent publication in the *Journal of Hospital Infection* seems to confirm the pilot study results. While the tea-tree oil product was not quite as good as mupirocin at reducing nasal colonisation with MRSA (although the difference was not statistically significant), the tea-tree oil skin wash performed better than a chlorhexidine wash. Our experience with tea-tree oil skin/body washes is that patients (and staff) generally prefer them to Triclosan or chlorhexidine. Tea-tree oil skin/body washes were recently shown to conform to a number of European Union guidelines for this type of product. Tea-tree oil preparations are only suitable for topical application; however, the use of topical conventional antibiotics is renowned for the promotion of resistance and the exploration of alternative agents such as tea-tree oil is certainly warranted.

As with many other 'natural' therapies, there have been concerns about safety, primarily in relation to skin sensitivity. While these issues are increasingly well-characterised, relatively limited data are available on the safety and toxicity of the oil.

> Anecdotal evidence from almost 80 years of use suggests that the topical use of tea-tree oil is relatively safe, and that adverse events are minor, self-limiting and occasional.

Published data indicate that tea-tree oil is toxic if ingested in higher doses and can also cause skin irritation at higher concentrations. Allergic reactions to tea-tree oil occur in predisposed individuals and may be due to the various oxidation products that are formed by exposure of the oil to light and/or air. Adverse reactions may be minimised by avoiding ingestion, applying only diluted oil topically and using oil that has been stored correctly. Data from individual components suggest that tea-tree oil has the potential to be developmentally toxic if ingested at higher doses; however, tea-tree oil and its components are not genotoxic. The limited ecotoxicity data available indicate that tea-tree oil is toxic to some insect species but more studies are required.

An important consideration for the efficacy of tea-tree oil (and other essential oils) is the composition of formulated products containing the active ingredient. Many excipients, and other components used to make cosmetic or pharmaceutical products, such as surfactants, can inactivate tea-tree oil and it is important to test any final product *in vitro* before embarking on clinical trials.

> There is now overwhelming evidence that essential oils such as tea-tree oil can play a role in the control of MRSA, although there is a need for further data on safety and clinical efficacy.

Garlic

Garlic (*Allium sativum*) was once used by millions to ward off vampires and was first used in around 3000 BC by the Sumerians, a group who still live in present day Iraq. Garlic has a wide spectrum of antimicrobial activity and is considered to be antibacterial, antiviral, antifungal and antiprotozoal. Although garlic has been used for its medicinal properties for thousands of years, investigations into its mode of action have occurred only relatively recently. Using a process of steam distillation, the German chemist Wertheim was able to obtain a pungent smelling oil from garlic cloves. Early steps in identifying the active constituents of garlic were the discovery that the compound allicin (allyl 2-propene thiosulphinate) is formed when garlic is crushed and that its formation depends on the action of the enzyme alliinase. Methyl and allyl sulphide derivatives of allicin are formed by the steam distillation of crushed garlic. The diallyl sulphide components of garlic oil are the most active and this activity is inversely proportional to the number of disulphide bonds, diallyl monosulphide having greatest activity. These diallyl sulphides inhibit various bacteria and fungi at concentrations similar to conventional antimicrobials. Several recent studies have shown good activity of garlic materials against *Helicobacter pylori* and clearly garlic has a long history of safe use. Epidemiological studies show a reciprocal relationship between gastric cancer, which is strongly correlated with *H. pylori* infection, and the consumption of *Allium* vegetables suggesting the further investigation of garlic as an antimicrobial is warranted.

> In relation to specific anti-MRSA activity, garlic extract given orally to mice infected with MRSA significantly reduced *in vivo* levels of MRSA, as well as inflammatory markers.

Honey

Honey has a long recorded history of medicinal use. Many reports can now be found in the medical literature describing the antibacterial properties of honey and honey products, and their potential as antimicrobial agents, particularly for wound care. Specific antibacterial activity has been described against a wide range of organisms, including MRSA; however, reported susceptibilities are not always consistent. Honey suffers from the same problems that most other 'natural' product research does in that honey from different botanical sources may differ in antimicrobial activity. The activity of honey has been attributed to the high osmolarity, the low pH and the presence of hydrogen peroxide, which is generated enzymatically. However, these factors alone or in combination do not account for all the antibacterial activity and there are additional phytochemical antibacterial factors that remain to be elucidated.

Bacteriophages as antimicrobial agents

An old idea ignored since the beginning of the antibiotic era by all but a few former Soviet block countries is bacteriophage therapy. Bacteriophage therapy for infectious diseases is not new. The idea was promulgated soon after the discovery of bacteriophages in the early 1900s and researched actively between 1920 and 1940. There has been renewed interest in bacteriophage therapy with the emergence of antibiotic-resistance as a major problem in modern medicine. Several reports from Poland in the 1980s described the treatment of various infections, the majority of which were staphylococcal. *In vitro* testing indicated that bacteriophage was active against specific pathogens. Efficacy *in vivo* was assessed on a clinical basis alone and positive results were obtained in over 90% of cases; however, there were no untreated controls.

Similar studies were carried out in the former Soviet Union from the early 1970s. In those studies where staphylococci (presumably *S. aureus*) were involved, bacteria were eliminated after phage therapy in the majority of cases. Phages were applied either topically, subcutaneously, or via irrigation or drains.

Studies originating in the UK have predominantly concentrated on the treatment of diarrhoeal disease, mainly caused by *Escherichia coli,* using animal models. However, bacteriophage successfully treated experimental *S. aureus* infections in mice but not when bacteriophage and *S. aureus* (the same strains as had been used in some of the Polish studies) were injected intraperitoneally, simultaneously. In this situation, bacteriophage was not protective although infections involving *Acinetobacter baumanii* and *Pseudomonas aeruginosa* could be prevented by their respective bacteriophages.

Several more recent reports offer an exciting glimpse of the potential of phage therapy. Intraperitoneal injection into mice of phage fMR11 suppressed *S. aureus,* including MRSA, lethality. High levels of the phage had no adverse effect on animals, and protection was evident even when mice were treated with phage 60 min after inoculation with bacteria. Abscess formation was prevented in a rabbit model of wound infection when phage was injected simultaneously with *S. aureus* into a subcutaneous site.

> Bacteriophage has been added to hand-wash solutions and used to obtain a 100-fold reduction in human skin staphylococci compared to a phage-free wash solution.

There have been several safety concerns about bacteriophage therapy. One has been the development of antiphage antibody during therapy. This was assessed in 57 patients following oral administration of bacteriophage and no measurable antibody was found in 44 during treatment. In two cases, high-titre antibody developed. Another major problem has been the presence of various toxins in crude phage lysates; however, this can now be addressed during preparative stages. The bioavailability of phage administered systemically has also been a concern, with early studies indicating that phage was quickly cleared by the reticulo-endothelial system.

Mutant phages with the ability to evade the reticulo-endothelial system have now been produced. It is possible that bacteria will ultimately became resistant to phage lysis in the same way that antibiotic resistance has emerged. However, the way in which phage would be used, as a single dose, would be less likely to result in resistance developing compared to antibiotics used over a long period. There may be other resistance problems, however, as some MRSA seem to be inherently less susceptible to bacteriophages than antibiotic-susceptible *S. aureus.* One final concern is the possibility of lysogenic conversion, whereby bacteriophage could acquire various toxin genes and introduce these into *S. aureus* strains. While a theoretical possibility, the likelihood of this occurring, or of virulence genes being introduced by transduction, is remote.

Bacterial interference

In the late 1960s and early 1970s, several papers from the US described the phenomenon of bacterial interference whereby some strains of *S. aureus* could prevent colonisation and/or infection with other strains. Bacterioprophylaxis was successful in halting an outbreak of virulent *S. aureus* infection among infants in a nursery and cases of chronic furunculosis. While the explanation for these successes could have been production of antagonistic compounds or competition for nutrients, the most likely mechanism is competitive adherence to specific attachment sites on host cells. Interest in this approach seems to have waned over the last 20 years, possibly due to ethics committees becoming somewhat nervous about introducing a live potential pathogen to an already compromised host. However, colonisation of the anterior nares with *S. aureus* is an important risk factor for *S. aureus* and MRSA infection, and a recent publication has revisited the relationship between methicillin-susceptible *S. aureus* (MSSA) and MRSA. The authors showed that MSSA was 78% effective in preventing MRSA colonisation of the nares. Hopefully this and an earlier publication that showed that viridans group streptococci could inhibit MRSA colonisation of the oral cavity in newborns will stimulate further work on this potentially useful approach.

Conclusions

Unfortunately, the medical profession has been slow to embrace natural or alternative therapies, and with good reason. Good scientific data are still scarce at present. However, as we approach the 'post-antibiotic era', the situation is changing. It behoves the informed practitioner to be aware of some of the possibilities and the current research status with these agents.

> 'Natural' therapies are viewed favourably by many patients, chiefly because they believe, often correctly, that they are associated with fewer detrimental effects than most antibiotics.

Further reading

Reviews

Carson CF, Hammer KA, Riley TV. *Melaleuca alternifolia* (tea tree) oil: a review of antimicrobial and other medicinal properties. *Clin Microbiol Rev* 2006; **19**: 50–62.

Carson CF, Riley TV. Non-antibiotic therapies for infectious diseases. *Comm Dis Intell* 2003; **27** *(Suppl)*: S144–7.

Cherwonogrodzky JW. Research strategies for the treatment of biothreats. *Curr Opin Pharmacol* 2005; **5**: 465–72.

Golledge CL, Riley TV. 'Natural' therapy for infectious diseases. *Med J Aust* 1996; **164**: 94–5.

Hammer KA, Carson CF, Riley TV, Nielsen JB. A review of the toxicity of *Melaleuca alternifolia* (tea tree) oil. *Food Chem Toxicol* 2006; In press.

Harris JC, Cottrell SL, Plummer S et al. Antimicrobial properties of *Allium sativum* (garlic). *Appl Microbiol Biotechnol* 2001; **57**: 282–6.

Mahady GB. Medicinal plants for the prevention and treatment of bacterial infections. *Curr Pharmacol Design* 2005; **11**: 2405–27.

Martin KW, Ernst E. Herbal medicines for treatment of bacterial infections: a review of controlled clinical trials. *J Antimicrob Chemother* 2003; **51**: 241–6.

Matzuzukii S, Rashel M, Uchiyama J et al. Bacteriophage therapy: a revitalized therapy against bacterial infectious diseases. *J Infect Chemother* 2005; **11**: 211–9.

Medicinal plants

Fukai T, Marumo A, Kaitou K et al. Antimicrobial activity of licorice flavonoids against methicillin-resistant *Staphylococcus aureus*. *Fitoterapia* 2002; **73**: 536–9.

Fukai T, Oku Y, Hano Y et al. Antimicrobial activities of hydrophobic 2-arylbenzofurans and an isoflavone against vancomycin-resistant *Enterococci* and methicillin-resistant *Staphylococcus aureus*. *Planta Med* 2004; **70**: 685–7.

Gibbons S, Leimkugel J, Oluwatuyi M et al. Activity of *Zanthoxylum clava-herculis* extracts against multi-drug resistant methicillin-resistant *Staphylococcus aureus* (mdr-MRSA). *Phytother Res* 2003; **17**: 274–5.

Gibbons S, Ohlendorf B, Johnsen I. The genus *Hypericum* – a valuable resource of anti-staphylococcal leads. *Fitoterapia* 2002; **73**: 300–4.

Hatano T, Kusuda M, Hori M et al. Theasinensin A, a tea polyphenol formed from (–)- epigallocatechin gallate, suppresses antibiotic resistance of methicillin-resistant *Staphylococcus aureus*. *Planta Med* 2003; **69**: 984–9.

Him K-J, Yu H-H, Cha J-D et al. Antibacterial activity of *Curcuma longa* L. against methicillin-resistant *Staphylococcus aureus*. *Phytother Res* 2005; **19**: 599–604.

Hur J-M, Yang C-H, Han S-H et al. Antibacterial effect of *Phellinus linteus* against methicillin-resistant *Staphylococcus aureus*. *Fitoterapia* 2004; **75**: 603–5.

Machado TB, Pinto Av, Pinto MCFR et al. *In vitro* activity of Brazilian medicinal plants, naturally occurring naphthoquinones and their analogues, against methicillin-resistant *Staphylococcus aureus*. *Int J Antimicrob Agents* 2003; **21**: 279–84.

Nishida S. Effect of Hochu-ekki-to on asymptomatic MRSA bacteriuria. *J Infect Chemother* 2003; **9**: 58–61.

Sakagami Y, Iinuma M, Piyasena KGNP et al. Antibacterial activity of α-mangostin against vancomycin resistant enterococci (VRE) and synergism with antibiotics. *Phytomedicine* 2005; **12**: 203–8.

Sato Y. Extraction and purification of effective antimicrobial constituents of *Terminalia chebula* Retz. against methicillin resistant *Staphylococcus aureus*. *Biol Pharmaceut Bull* 1997; **20**: 410–4.

Smith, E, Williamson E, Zloh M et al. Isopimaric acid from *Pinus nigra* shows activity against multidrug-resistant and EMRSA strains of *Staphylococcus aureus*. *Phytother Res* 2005; **19**: 538–42.

Tanaka H, Sato M, Oh-Uchi T et al. Antibacterial properties of a new isoflavonoid from *Erythrina poeppigiana* against methicillin-resistant *Staphylococcus aureus*. *Phytomedicine* 2004; **11**: 331–7.

Essential oils

Edwards-Jones V, Buck R, Shawcross SG et al. The effect of essential oils on methicillin-resistant *Staphylococcus aureus* using a dressing model. *Burns* 2004; **30**: 772–7.

Hammer KA, Carson CF, Riley TV. Antimicrobial activity of essential oils and other plant extracts. *J Appl Microbiol* 1999; **86**: 985–90.

Lis-Balchin M, Hart SL, Deans SG. Pharmacological and antimicrobial studies on different tea-tree oils (*Melaleuca alternifolia, Leptospermum scoparium* or Manuka and *Kunzea ericoides* or Kanuka), originating in Australia and New Zealand. *Phytother Res* 2000; **14**: 623–9.

Matsunaga T, Hasegawa C, Kawasuji T *et al.* Isolation of the antiulcer compound in essential oil from the leaves of *Cryptomeria japonica. Biol Pharm Bull* 2000; **23**: 595–8.

Porter NG, Wilkins AL. Chemical, physical and antimicrobial properties of essential oils of *Leptospermum scoparium* and *Kunzea ericoides. Phytochemistry* 1998; **50**: 407–15.

Skocibusic M, Bezic N. Phytochemical analysis and *in vitro* antimicrobial activity of two *Satureja* species essential oils. *Phytother Res* 2004; **18**: 967–70.

Tea-tree oil

Anderson JN, Fennessy PA. Can tea tree (*Melaleuca alternifolia*) oil prevent MRSA? *Med J Aust* 2000; **173**: 489.

Caelli M, Porteous J, Carson CF *et al.* Tea tree oil as an alternative topical decolonization agent for methicillin-resistant *Staphylococcus aureus. J Hosp Infect* 2000; **46**: 236–7.

Carson CF, Cookson BD, Farrelly HD *et al.* Susceptibility of methicillin-resistant *Staphylococcus aureus* to the essential oil of *Melaleuca alternifolia. J Antimicrob Chemother* 1995; **35**: 421–4.

Carson CF, Riley TV. Antimicrobial activity of the major components of the essential oil of *Melaleuca alternifolia. J Appl Bacteriol* 1995; **78**: 264–9.

Carson CF, Riley TV, Cookson BD. Efficacy and safety of tea tree oil as a topical antimicrobial agent. *J Hosp Infect* 1998; **40**: 175–8.

Carson CF, Mee BJ, Riley TV. Mechanism of action of *Melaleuca alternifolia* (tea tree) oil on *Staphylococcus aureus* determined by time-kill, lysis, leakage, and salt tolerance assays and electron microscopy. *Antimicrob Agents Chemother* 2002; **46**: 1914–20.

Dryden MS, Dailly AS, Crouch M. A randomized, controlled trial of tea tree topical preparations versus a standard topical regimen for the clearance of MRSA colonization. *J Hosp Infect* 2004; **56**: 283–6.

Flaxman D, Griffiths P. Is tea tree oil effective at eradicating MRSA colonization? *Br J Community Nur* 2005; **10**: 123–6.

Halcon L, Milkus BA. *Staphylococcus aureus* and wounds: a review of tea tree oil as a promising antimicrobial. *Am J Infect Control* 2004; **32**: 402–8.

Hammer KA, Carson CF, Riley TV. Susceptibility of transient and commensal skin flora to the essential oil of *Melaleuca alternifolia* (tea tree oil). *Am J Infect Control* 1996; **24**: 186–9.

Hammer KA, Carson CF, Riley TV. Influence of organic matter, cations and surfactants on the antimicrobial activity of *Melaleuca alternifolia* (tea tree) oil *in vitro. J Appl Microbiol* 1999; **86**: 446–52.

May J, Chan CH, King A *et al.* Time-kill studies of tea tree oils on clinical isolates. *J Antimicrob Chemother* 2000; **45**: 639–43.

Messager S, Hammer KA, Carson CF, Riley TV. Effectiveness of hand cleansing formulations containing tea tree oil assessed *ex-vivo*, on human skin, and *in-vivo* with volunteers using European standard EN 1499. *J Hosp Infect* 2005; **59**: 220–8.

Messager S, Hammer KA, Carson CF, Riley TV. Assessment of the antibacterial activity of tea tree oil using the European EN 1276 and EN 12054 standard suspension tests. *J Hosp Infect* 2005; **59**: 113–25.

Garlic

O'Gara EA, Hill DJ, Maslin DJ. Activities of garlic oil, garlic powder, and their diallyl constituents against *Helicobacter pylori. Appl Environ Microbiol* 2000; **66**: 2269–73.

Tsao S-M, Yin M-C. *In-vitro* antimicrobial activity of four diallyl sulphides occurring naturally in garlic and Chinese leek oils. *J Med Microbiol* 2001; **50**: 646–9.

Tsao S-M, Hsu C-c, Yin Mei-chin. Garlic extract and two diallyl sulphides inhibit methicillin-resistant *Staphylococcus aureus* infection in BALB/cA mice. *J Antimicrob Chemother* 2003; **52**: 974–80.

Honey

Cooper RA, Molan PC, Harding KG. The sensitivity to honey of Gram-positive cocci of clinical significance isolated from wounds. *J Appl Microbiol* 2002; **93**: 857–63.

Molan PC. The antibacterial activity of honey. 1. The nature of the antibacterial activity. *Bee World* 1992; **73**: 5–28.

Molan PC. The antibacterial activity of honey. 2. Variations in the potency of the antibacterial activity. *Bee World* 1992; **73**: 59–76.

Bacteriophage therapy

Alisky J, Iczkowski K, Rapoport A *et al.* Bacteriophages show promise as antimicrobial agents. *J Infect* 1998; **36**: 5–15.

Bruttin A, Brussow H. Human volunteers receiving *Escherichia coli* phage T4 orally: a safety test of phage therapy. *Antimicrob Agents Chemother* 2005; **49**: 2874–8.

Matsuda T, Freeman TA, Hilbert DW *et al.* Lysis-deficient bacteriophage therapy decreases endotoxin and inflammatory mediator release and improves survival in a murine peritonitis model. *Surgery* 2005; **137**: 639–46.

Matsuzaki S, Yasuda M, Nishikawa H *et al.* Experimental protection of mice against lethal *Staphylococcus aureus* infection by novel bacteriophage fMR11. *J Infect Dis* 2003; **187**: 613–24.

Merrill CR, Biswas B, Carlton R *et al*. Long-circulating bacteriophage as antibacterial agents. *Proc Natl Acad Sci USA* 1996; **93**: 3188–92.

O'Flaherty S, Ross RP, Meaney W *et al*. Potential of the polyvalent anti-*Staphylococcus* bacteriophage K for control of antibiotic-resistant staphylococci from hospitals. *Appl Environ Microbiol* 2005; **71**: 1836–42.

Parfitt T. Georgia: an unlikely stronghold for bacteriophage therapy. *Lancet* 2005; **365**: 2166–7.

Sau K, Gupta SK, Sau S *et al*. Synonymous codon usage bias in 16 *Staphylococcus aureus* phages: implication in phage therapy. *Virus Res* 2005; **113**: 123–31.

Soothill JS. Treatment of experimental infections of mice with bacteriophages. *J Med Microbiol* 1992; **37**: 258–61.

Sulakvelidze A. Phage therapy: an attractive option for dealing with antibiotic-resistant bacterial infections. *Drug Discovery Today* 2005; **10**: 808–9.

Wills QF, Kerrigan C, Soothill JS. Experimental bacteriophage protection against *Staphylococcus aureus* abscesses in a rabbit model. *Antimicrob Agents Chemother* 2005; **49**: 1220–1.

Bacterial interference

Aly R, Maibach HI, Shinefield N *et al*. Bacterial interference among strains of *Staphylococcus aureus* in man. *J Infect Dis* 1974; **129**: 720–4.

Bibel DJ, Aly R, Bayles C *et al*. Competitive adherence as a mechanism of bacterial interference. *Can J Microbiol* 1983; **29**: 700–3.

Dall'Antonia M, Coen PG, Wilks M *et al*. Competition between methicillin-sensitive and –resistant *Staphylococcus aureus* in the anterior nares. *J Hosp Infect* 2005; **61**: 62–7.

Light IJ, Walton RL, Sutherland JM *et al*. Use of bacterial interference to control a staphylococcal nursery outbreak. *Am J Dis Child* 1967; **113**: 291–300.

Maibach HI, Strauss WG, Shinefield HR. Bacterial interference: relating to chronic furunculosis in man. *Br J Dermatol* 1969; **81 (Suppl 1)**: 69–76.

Rao GG, Wong J. Interaction between methicillin-resistant *Staphylococcus aureus* (MRSA) and methicillin-sensitive *Staphylococcus aureus* (MSSA). *J Hosp Infect* 2003; **55**: 116–8.

Uehara Y, Kikuchi K, Nakamura T *et al*. Inhibition of methicillin-resistant *Staphylococcus aureus* colonization of oral cavities in newborn by viridans group streptococci. *Clin Infect Dis* 2001; **32**: 1399–407.

13. Mopping up MRSA

Stephanie J Dancer

Background
History of staphylococcal epidemiology
Staphylococcal transmission cycle
Staphylococcal carriage
Airborne transmission
Contamination in hospitals
Survival of staphylococci
Human transmission
Dynamic relationship
Effect of cleaning
Importance of hand-touch sites

There is no scientific evidence to support cleaning as a valid control mechanism for MRSA and other hospital-acquired pathogens in hospitals

There is an on-going debate about the importance of hospital cleaning in relation to the increasing numbers of patients acquiring methicillin-resistant *Staphylococcus aureus* (MRSA). It is possible that basic cleaning might help us to control such pathogens but there is currently no scientific evidence for this in hospitals. Since a clean environment has always been taken for granted, perhaps it is not surprising that there is no evidence for cleanliness as a significant control factor in the spread of MRSA. In addition, we have no way of measuring how clean a hospital is other than a visual assessment. This is both subjective and inaccurate, given that such an assessment does not necessarily correlate with microbiological risk. We cannot see MRSA in the environment and we certainly do not know exactly how it is transmitted to patients in hospitals. At present, only aesthetic demands from patients and their relatives appear to support the removal of dirt in hospitals.

Background

Several professional bodies have published standards or audits for the express purpose of improving the appearance of the hospital environment and thus helping to alleviate public concern. There have also been NHS cleaning manuals, model cleaning contracts and monitoring strategies. Unfortunately, these utilise nothing more than a visual assessment and fail to recognise the fact that micro-organisms, including human pathogens, are invisible to the naked eye. The Department of Health itself has stated that: 'Clean hospitals are about the cleanliness of the floors, clean linen and clean toilets – that doesn't affect MRSA rates'. Clean-looking hospitals may well help to restore public confidence and staff morale in the short-term, but will not necessarily reduce the rate of acquisition of MRSA.

In addition, the lack of scientific evidence leaves the cleaning process vulnerable to cost-cutting exercises by NHS managers. Consequently, the number of cleaners has halved over the last decade. Cleaners are not the best-paid staff in a hospital, and removing dirt and debris is not afforded the status it deserves. There is little support for what they do, and this is manifest in high sickness rates, lack of training, poor equipment, high turnover and job dissatisfaction. It is also the case that cleaning is hard work, and hospital cleaning itself is a speciality in its own right. It is far more difficult to clean a hospital ward than an office or supermarket. Cleaners in hospital are also more at risk of contracting an infection, since they are regularly exposed to hospital pathogens. Evidence for cleaning would increase their status, generate accompanying benefits, and might help alleviate the present workforce situation.

History of staphylococcal epidemiology

Cleaning aesthetics aside, there are a few studies that suggest that cleaning helps to reduce the risk of acquiring MRSA in hospitals. They are far from conclusive, however, because the cleaning component is never studied in isolation from other control factors. There has to be another way of validating cleaning as a potential control strategy for MRSA. From the work of the staphylococcal pioneers 50 years ago, we already have evidence to support all the individual components of the staphylococcal transmission cycle between patients, staff and the inanimate environment. Each component of this transmission cycle can be considered independently in order to assess the impact of removing MRSA from the environment. Much of the early work on the properties of the coagulase-positive staphylococcus is as relevant today, with MRSA, as it was with the 'hospital staph' of the 1950s and 1960s. The epidemiological properties of *S. aureus*, whether methicillin resistant or not, remain the same.

The main difference between the 'hospital staph' 50 years ago and present strains of MRSA is that isoxazolyl penicillins (*e.g.* flucloxacillin) quickly and easily treated patients with infections caused by *S. aureus* before it could be spread to others, or dispersed throughout the hospital environment. We do not have a 'flucloxacillin' for MRSA – the drugs we do have are toxic, expensive, and relatively inefficient and most have to be given parenterally. Patients with low-grade infection or colonisation with MRSA tend to be managed conservatively, thus enhancing their own risk for future invasive sepsis. They are also more likely to shed the organism into the environment as well as spread it to other patients and staff. This lends support for cleaning as a possible control factor. Hospital wards were also a lot cleaner in the 1950s and 1960s; they had not been exposed to today's penny-pinching managers and the removal of dirt received a higher priority. There has been a gradual erosion of the importance of hygiene in our society, emanating from the provision of antimicrobial agents.

Staphylococcal transmission cycle

Humans carry coagulase-positive staphylococci and disperse the bacteria into the environment. People may pick up the bacteria from the environment but can also acquire *S. aureus* from others directly, generally by touch. About 30% of the population are found to carry *S. aureus* at any one time; this includes 20% who always seem to be colonised, and a further 10% who fall into a transient carriage group.

Coagulase-positive staphylococci may be found colonising people, in the surrounding air, in the environment in which they live, or through which they have just passed. Given the propensity for people to pick, touch or blow their noses, it is not surprising that habitual carriers will often demonstrate their own strain of *S. aureus* on fingers, which they will then transfer to any site accessible for hand touch.

In addition, all of the members of the staphylococcal family – coagulase-negative and -positive – demonstrate an avid ability to survive in the environment, throughout a wide range of temperatures, humidity, exposure to sunlight and desiccation. This increases the chance that someone will acquire viable staphylococci from the environment, since the organism awaits its opportunity to be picked up and transferred or inoculated into a new host.

There is thus a dynamic staphylococcal transmission cycle between man and his environment, perpetuating the survival of this generally human commensal (Fig. 13.1). Given these properties, it is apparent that there are a number of stages representing all the possible scenarios relating to transmission. These can be broken down into individual statements, for which can be found evidence, and which taken together, demonstrate the potential for an environmental role in staphylococcal acquisition and consequently, support for cleaning.

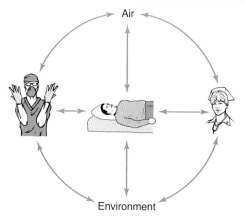

Figure 13.1
Staphylococcal transmission cycle

Staphylococcal carriage

S. aureus colonises multiple body sites of humans, of which the anterior nares is the most frequent carriage site. There appears to be an inherent capacity for some people to carry *S. aureus*, in that certain individuals habitually carry *S. aureus* in the nose and recolonise very quickly following eradication attempts. They may carry the same strain for months, or even years, unless it is replaced by another strain displaying greater adhesive properties. Specific strains appear to be so attached to their human host that they can almost be said to resemble the territorial nature of robins in the back garden. Screening exercises amongst the normal population do not usually identify more than one strain colonising a habitual carrier.

There is a link between *S. aureus* nasal carriage and staphylococcal infection. A causal relation between carriage and an infecting strain is demonstrated by the fact that the nasal strain of *S. aureus* and the infecting strain often share the same genotype. Application of a topical antibiotic into the nose temporarily eliminates carriage and reduces the risk of infection.

The extent to which a carrier sheds his or her strain into the environment is very variable. Some are surrounded by minute skin particles associated with a few colony-forming units of staphylococci in such great quantities that they are referred to as a 'cloud adult'. This is seen in people suffering an upper respiratory tract infection or those with exfoliative skin conditions. Some shed following antibiotic treatment; some depending upon which sites are colonised and others appear never to shed at all.

> Some strains of *S. aureus* stick to nasal epithelium so well, that they resist replacement by other strains and thus resemble the territorial nature of robins in the back garden.

Airborne transmission

Air sampling, settle plates and environmental microbiological screening are among the methods used to locate coagulase-positive staphylococci in the general environment. Skin particles with adherent staphylococci fall to the floor under the influence of gravity, or indeed onto any horizontal surface interrupting their flight. Thus, air sampling demonstrates the dynamic nature of staphylococcal dispersal but the final common resting place is usually the floor. Air currents or draughts, such as created when a door or window is opened, will encourage skin particles to remain air-borne; equally, a sudden blast of air will elevate resting particles to become air-borne once again. Smaller and generally more mobile particles will take longer to sink to the ground and are, therefore, more susceptible to air turbulence.

Various studies have specifically investigated the presence of MRSA in air in hospitals. One carried out a sequence of air sampling before and after bed making and showed that MRSA counts remained elevated for up to 15 minutes after bed making was complete. It follows that if airborne transmission of MRSA is a significant risk for acquisition, more patients in a relatively small confined space will increase the likelihood of predisposing a patient to initial colonisation. Certainly, increased bed numbers have been shown to correlate with an increased risk of MRSA colonisation.

Contamination in hospitals

The evidence for both S. aureus and MRSA contamination of a huge variety of items in hospitals is overwhelming. Objects such as door handles, tourniquets, pens, computer keyboards, television sets, stethoscopes, telephones, beds and bedside tables, sterile goods' packaging, paper and patient's notes, toys and clinical equipment are just a few examples. The fact that most of these items are hand-touch objects should also be mentioned when considering the origin of the MRSA contamination. If staphylococcal carriers are likely to carry their resident strain on fingers, it stands to reason that anything that depends upon hands for functionality is at risk of acquiring a carrier's strain, although subsequent persistence would be dependent upon additional factors. It is also fair to say that an habitual carrier is not necessarily required to transfer MRSA to hand-touch objects, since anyone who has just touched a contaminated site would be able to do the same.

> MRSA has been isolated from numerous articles in hospitals as well as throughout the general environment. Specific items known to harbour MRSA include door handles, bedside lockers, blood-pressure cuffs, patients' notes, nurse call-buttons, telephones, pens, doctors' ties, computers, curtains, stethoscopes and children's toys

Laundered items and soft furnishings are also at risk for contamination and there are plenty of reports detailing MRSA from bedclothes, pillows, mattresses and cushions. Nurses' uniforms and doctors' ties have also been implicated, with predictable media response generated by the latter. Ward curtains have long been suspected as capable of harbouring staphylococci. Studies from the 1960s showed that S. aureus could be isolated from ward curtains beside a patient with a staphylococcal infection, and that the two isolates demonstrated the same phage type. The important point about curtains is that they are often the first object touched after examining a patient on the ward round – even before the examining doctor or nurse has had a chance to wash their hands. Furthermore, the difficulties entailed by removing them for cleaning will, in today's fraught NHS, condemn them to remain in place for much longer than is desirable. Off-site laundries, bed pressures and shortage of spare curtains and the space to put them, all compound the management of ward curtains. Replacing them with vertical blinds will not alleviate these problems, since these are just as likely to become contaminated and may be even more difficult to clean.

Survival of staphylococci

Staphylococci are quite capable of surviving long-term in the environment, whether it is in the hospital, the home or, indeed, in any public place. Its resistance to desiccation is long established and persistence is easily demonstrated by any microbiological laboratory. There is little difference between the survival properties demonstrated by S. aureus and its methicillin-resistant version, although there appear to be differences in survival times between sporadic and epidemic resistant strains. Epidemic strains, as might be expected, do seem to be able to survive better than their sporadic counterparts in hospital dust. Otherwise, there are plenty of reports describing survival of MRSA on articles ranging from paper to mops, to more general studies examining persistence on Formica, hospital fabrics and plastics. Even deep cleaning a ward using detergent and a steam cleaner, followed by 1000-ppm chlorine disinfectant for all hard surfaces, does not completely eradicate MRSA from the clinical environment. This persistence adds to the support for cleaning in the removal of MRSA from hospitals, although it is possible that we are not using the best methods in UK hospitals at present.

Human transmission

We know that healthcare staff can acquire MRSA from positive patients and/or their environment. It was thought that contamination of a physician's office was responsible for subsequent recolonisation, following apparently successful topical clearance in one case. In hospital, just less than half of the nurses entering the rooms of MRSA patients acquire the patient's strain of MRSA on gloved hands and aprons. Nearly two-thirds of nurses will acquire the organism if they have direct contact with the patient.

Other work has shown that about 17% contacts between a healthcare worker and an MRSA-colonised patient result in transmission of MRSA from the patient to the gloves of the healthcare worker. An additional study examined the frequency of acquisition of various pathogens, including MRSA, on investigators' hands after contacting environmental surfaces near hospitalised patients. About 30% of hand imprint cultures yielded coagulase-positive staphylococci from the bed rail and bedside table in occupied rooms, although only half of the patients were known to have prior colonisation or infection with *S. aureus* or MRSA.

There are further reports detailing staphylococcal transmission between humans in hospitals and at home. These relate to outbreak situations involving healthcare workers or patients newly transferred from elsewhere. Others describe transmission from healthcare workers to family members, spread between patients in the community and transmission between ambulant patients.

> Persistent staphylococcal carriage may be associated with contamination of the home environment or unidentified carriage by a family member

It could be said that the evidence for human-to-human transmission is of less relevance regarding environmental contamination with MRSA and its amelioration by cleaning, in that the demonstration of such transmission effectively negates the importance of MRSA in the environment and its removal. Whilst there

is no doubt that carriers can transmit their strain to others, none of the studies mentioned specify, or provide evidence, for the exact mechanism of this transfer. Thus it may be assumed that indirect transmission via the environment is as likely as direct person-to-person transmission. At least two studies have shown that staphylococcal carriage is associated with contamination of the home environment, and that refractory carriage may be attributed to the presence of MRSA in the home environment.

Dynamic relationship between people and the environment regarding staphylococcal transmission

Many studies have demonstrated the presence of coagulase-positive staphylococci throughout the hospital environment. Furthermore, some studies have established that environmental strains may be genotypically indistinguishable from strains obtained from patients within the same environment. One of these showed related strains from staff, patients and the environment. There appears to be an indisputable relationship between people and their environments regarding staphylococcal transmission, but we do not know from where the strains originated, or in which direction they travelled. A 4-month study in an intensive care unit collected coagulase-negative staphylococci from staff hands, ITU environment and patients' blood. It found that indistinguishable strains could be identified from all three sources within a relatively short time frame. Whilst coagulase-negative staphylococci do not usually demonstrate the same pathogenic potential as *S. aureus* and MRSA, they do share similar epidemiology and could be said to act as an indicator for their more pathogenic counterparts.

> Fingerprinting staphylococcal isolates confirms indistinguishable strains from staff hands, patients' blood and environmental sites in the hospital.

Effect of cleaning

There are only a handful of studies that suggest that cleaning is useful in the event of an outbreak of MRSA. A concerted effort in the early 1970s to rid a district general hospital of MRSA was successful, utilising a programme of ward closure, cleaning, increased screening and other infection control interventions. The overall rate of *S. aureus* infections also decreased significantly. More recently, there has been one study only, where the usual infection control activities had no effect on an MRSA epidemic among male surgical patients until the time allocated for basic cleaning of the ward was doubled. Following this, the outbreak strain was eliminated from the ward environment and there were no more infections among the patients with this particular strain. This study is also notable for attempting to calculate the cost/benefit of the cleaning intervention; this was estimated as nearly £28,000 for the 6 months when the extra cleaning took place. The authors categorically concluded that in the long term, cost cutting on cleaning services is neither cost-effective nor common sense.

A number of studies detailing cleaning methods have appeared recently. These include routine vacuuming and detergent-based cleaning, deep cleaning with disinfectants and gaseous decontamination using hydrogen peroxide vapour. All appear to reduce MRSA in the hospital environment, although a standardised measurement of bacterial counts was not employed. A move towards quantitation of bacterial load in the hospital environment is becoming more evident, with a proposal for standards for surface-level cleanliness in hospitals as a baseline for further work on the efficacy of various cleaning methods. So many of the recent standards for hospital hygiene recommend the use of 'visual cleanliness' as a performance criterion, yet it is known that visually clean surfaces may not be microbiologically or chemically clean.

> There has been a recent proposal to adopt microbiological standards in the assessment of hospital cleanliness.

Importance of near-patient, hand-touch sites

Perhaps there is another way to tackle the presence of MRSA in our hospitals other than campaigning for more cleaning hours. We know that visual appearance is an unreliable guide to the presence of pathogenic microbes. Perhaps targeting the areas in a hospital that constitute the highest risk for the presence of MRSA would be a feasible option in the short-term. Buffing the floors in out-patient departments might improve the appearance of the waiting areas, but patients do not generally acquire MRSA from floors. The greatest risk for patients is contaminated near-patient, hand-touch sites in clinical areas and it is these sites that should be targeted for extra cleaning attention.

Ward cleaners work to a set specification that does not necessarily include near-patient, hand-touch sites. Responsibility for cleaning these more often rests with the ward nurses, who are often very busy and currently in short supply in UK hospitals. A recent study in an intensive care unit demonstrated an increased risk of MRSA clusters following periods of inadequate nurse staffing. These clusters also appeared to be associated with hygiene failures, which were identified at the same time as the nursing shortages. In addition, another study has confirmed that there are high rates of cleaning of traditional sites, such as toilet surfaces and sinks, but poor cleaning of many sites that have significant potential for harbouring and transmitting microbial pathogens. These sites include handles, doorknobs and handholds. It may be that concentrating available cleaning resources on high-risk hand-touch sites would be the most cost-effective strategy at the present time.

> Concentrating cleaning resources on near-patient, hand-touch sites might be more cost-effective than buffing floors in out-patient areas.

> Any benefits from washing your hands are eroded if the environment is heavily contaminated with MRSA.

Conclusions

Common sense tells us that reducing the numbers of microbes on an object or in the general environment should not only reduce the risk of there being a pathogen present, but ought to reduce the risk of infection for persons in contact with that object or environment. Unfortunately, 'common sense' is unable to justify additional managerial spending upon the domestic budget unless there is clear evidence of benefit. At present, we just do not have that evidence. The increasing prevalence of MRSA and other multiply-resistant bacteria in UK hospitals, however, justify cleaning and other control measures ahead of their definitive validation.

Most people think that hand decontamination is far more important than cleaning in a hospital. There can be no doubt that hand hygiene is the single most beneficial intervention regarding the control of MRSA and numerous other pathogens. The problem with hand hygiene, however, is that it is impossible to get everyone to do it at the most appropriate time. In any case, the effects of exemplary hand hygiene are eroded if the environment is heavily contaminated with MRSA. We actually need both together if we are to see any improvement in the current acquisition rate of MRSA in UK hospitals.

Cleaners are not valued as they should be and their salaries reflect this. It is beyond belief that more cleaning hours cannot be squeezed out of the NHS budget, particularly when there is evidence for significant savings. Cost of drugs alone to treat a patient with an MRSA infection justifies the immediate prioritisation of domestic resources in clinical areas.

Further reading

Anon. *NHS Cleaning Manual*. London: Department of Health, 2004.

Boyce JM. Environmental contamination due to methicillin-resistant *Staphylococcus aureus*: possible infection control implications. *Infect Control Hosp Epidemiol* 1997; **18**: 622–7.

Dancer SJ. How do we assess hospital cleaning? A proposal for microbiological standards for surface hygiene in hospitals. *J Hosp Infect* 2004; **56**: 10–5.

Griffith CJ, Cooper RA, Gilmore J, Davies C, Lewis M. An evaluation of hospital cleaning regimes and standards. *J Hosp Infect* 2000; **45**: 19–28.

Lidwell OM. Some aspects of transfer and acquisition of *Staphylococcus aureus* in hospitals. In: Macdonald A, Smith G. (eds) *The Staphylococci*. Proceedings of the Alexander Ogston Centennial Conference. Aberdeen: Aberdeen University Press, 1981.

Noone P, Griffiths RJ. The effect of sepsis rates of closing and cleaning hospital wards. *J Clin Pathol* 1971; **24**: 721–5.

Rampling A, Wiseman S, Davis L *et al*. Evidence that hospital hygiene is important in the control of methicillin-resistant *Staphylococcus aureus*. *J Hosp Infect* 2001; **49**: 109–16.

Wertheim HFL, Melles DC, Vos MC *et al*. The role of nasal carriage in *Staphylococcus aureus* infections. *Lancet Infect Dis* 2005; **5**: 751–62.

14. MRSA control in the community

Hans Jørn Kolmos

Epidemiology
Aim and strategy
Detection of MRSA
Nursing homes and other long-term
    care facilities
Clients receiving home care
Schools, kindergartens and day-care
    centres
Clinics
Ambulances, taxis and public
    transport
Treatment of MRSA carriers and
    follow-up

Epidemiology

MRSA is detected with increasing frequency in patients outside hospitals.[1,2] In a recent meta-analysis, the overall prevalence of MRSA colonisation in community members was 1.3%, with great variation among study populations.[3]

The majority of cases were not really community-acquired, but originated from patients, who had recently been hospitalised or had other risk factors for acquisition of MRSA. The prevalence of truly community-acquired MRSA, i.e. MRSA in patients without risk factors, did not exceed 0.2%.[3]

MRSA may spread everywhere in the community, where people are in physical contact and share equipment and facilities, such as rest rooms and changing rooms. Transmission of MRSA has been reported in nursing homes and other long-term care facilities,[4,5] prisons and military camps,[6,7] sports clubs,[8] schools and kindergartens,[9] work places,[9] and semi-closed societies of ethnic minorities.[2,9] Transmission may also take place in households with a known MRSA carrier.[3] Persons with wounds, chronic skin disorders, chronic sinusitis, and in-dwelling catheters run a particularly high risk for colonisation with MRSA. Table 14.1 summarises the groups with increased risk for acquisition and transmission of MRSA. MRSA carriers, who are colonised in the nose and upper respiratory tract, may be particularly contagious in connection viral respiratory tract infections ('cloud persons').[10]

Until recently, MRSA was not considered a problem outside hospitals. Strains originating from hospitals are usually multiresistant and, therefore, not particularly fit for long-term survival in the community, where the selection pressure from antibiotics is much lower and the antibiotic consumption pattern is different. Furthermore, due to attenuated virulence,

Table 14.1
Risk factors for acquisition of MRSA in community members

Risk situations
- Residence in, or recent admission to, nursing homes and other long-term care facilities
- Recent hospitalisation or out-patient visits
- Recent antibiotic exposure
- Present or recent stay in prisons and other correctional facilities
- Intravenous drug abuse
- Close contact with person known to be MRSA positive, or with risk factors for MRSA acquisition

Risk-associated illnesses
- Chronic illness with high risk for staphylococcal carriage (e.g. diabetes and end-stage kidney disease)
- Chronic wounds (e.g. leg and foot ulcers, pressure sores)
- Chronic skin diseases (e.g. eczema and psoriasis)
- Chronic respiratory tract diseases
- In-dwelling catheters
- Recent surgery

hospital-acquired MRSA strains are rarely pathogenic to healthy individuals, and the potential for contact transmission in the community is much lower than in hospitals.

Unfortunately, this situation is in the process of change. In recent years, MRSA clones have emerged that are particularly fit for survival and spread in the community.[1,11] These clones characteristically contain virulence genes, which enhance their ability to become invasive and cause severe infections in previously healthy individuals. Examples of such genes are the Panton-Valentine leukocidin (PVL) toxin genes, which produce cytotoxins that can cause tissue necrosis and leukocyte destruction. In contrast to hospital-acquired MRSA strains, which are usually multidrug resistant, these new clones as a rule contain only few acquired resistance characters, often they are only mono-β-lactam resistant. This implies that they are not dependent on a heavy antibiotic selection pressure to favour their spread. Furthermore, the gene cassette mediating resistance (SSCmec type) is quite small, and at the same time provided with functional integrase genes. This implies that it can easily be packed in phages and transferred horizontally to other staphylococcal strains and integrated in their genomes. Some of these strains may have special virulence characters; in this way, new MRSA clones may emerge that are particularly fit to spread and cause disease in the previously healthy people in the community. An example of such a clone is the PVL positive ST80 SCCmectype IV clone, which has been reported from countries all over Europe.[12] Table 14.2 summarises the more important differences between hospital-acquired and community-acquired MRSA strains.

Although the vast majority of MRSA carriers in the community remain asymptomatic, it is evident that these new and more virulent clones give rise to increasing morbidity, even in previously healthy individuals. The most common types of infections are skin and soft-tissue infections, such as impetigo, furuncles and boils.[11–13] However, more severe conditions, such as necrotising fasciitis and necrotising pneumonia has also been reported.[14,15] Furthermore, recent studies indicate that these clones can also be introduced and spread in hospitals, where they may give rise to severe conditions, such as prosthetic joint infections and postpartum infections.[16,17]

So, we are facing a new epidemiological situation with community-associated MRSA. The main issue is no longer a displacement of

Table 14.2
Comparison of traditional hospital-acquired MRSA and new emerging community-acquired strains

Strain characteristics	Hospital-acquired MRSA	Community-acquired MRSA
Genetic origin	5 major global clones	Different genetic backgrounds, presumably due to horizontal transfer of resistance genes
Antibiotic resistance		
• SSCmec types	I, II, III	IV
• Motility and promiscuity of resistance genes	Low	High
• Phenotypic profile	Usually multidrug resistant	Usually mono β-lactam resistant
Virulence factors		
• PVL-producing	Few strains	Most strains
• Other toxins	Fewer	More
Major clinical presentation	Surgical wound infections and device-associated infections	Primary wound and soft-tissue infections

SSC, staphylococcal cassette chromosome; PVL, Panton-Valentine leukocidin.

hospital-acquired MRSA strains to the community with low risk for spread and disease, but the emergence of new and more virulent strains well adapted to community settings, and with a proven capability to disseminate and cause severe infections even in previously healthy individuals. Furthermore, if these strains get a foothold in hospitals and merge with existing MRSA strains this could result in the emergence of new multiresistant strains with enhanced virulence. Thus, control of MRSA in the community is of great importance, not only for community members, but in the long run also for hospitalised patients. This calls for enforcement of the containment strategies used up till now in community settings.

Aim and strategy

The emergence of MRSA strains which have a potential for spread in the community necessitates extra effort to avoid these strains from becoming endemic. The overall aim is to keep community-acquired MRSA at the lowest possible level and avoid strain introduction and spread in hospitals, nursing homes and other long-term care facilities.

Since most cases are asymptomatic, MRSA cannot be controlled by specific measures alone. General precautions focusing on the prevention of contact transmission make up the basic principle for control of MRSA. The major general precautions are:

- hand hygiene
- use of personal protective means including gloves, gowns and aprons, if relevant
- safe procedures for processing of laundry and disposal of waste
- decontamination of equipment
- good standards for domestic cleaning, with focus on keeping the environment free of dust.

Hand hygiene is the most important single factor for containment of MRSA, but despite its importance it is often neglected. Therefore,

special efforts should be made to introduce good hand-hygiene practices in all community settings. Training programmes should focus not only on frequencies of hand hygiene, but also on good hand-hygiene techniques.[18,19] In particular, the use of alcoholic hand rubs should be encouraged. Managers should ensure that proper facilities for hand washing (sinks, soap and paper towels) are easily available.

In addition to these basic principles, it is necessary to add a number of specific precautions, once MRSA has been detected. Specific precautions tailored for different community settings are outlined below.

Detection of MRSA

Containment of MRSA in the community, as well as in hospitals, is dependent on the ability to recognise cases.

> Detection of MRSA can only be done by laboratory testing, irrespective of whether patients are infected or colonised. It is, therefore, essential that primary healthcare services have free access to microbiological testing in the same way as hospitals, and that doctors make use of it.

Special attention should be paid to patients with risk factors (Table 14.1), and to skin and soft-tissue infections in children and previously healthy adults, particularly if cases tend to cluster. Screening for MRSA carriage may give rise to much anxiety, and implies a risk of stigmatisation of those who are tested positive.

> Screening should only be done if there is a qualified suspicion of MRSA and if there is a clear plan of how to deal with individuals who are tested positive. Broad-scale testing without a plan is a waste of resources and may do more harm than good.

The proportions of screening for MRSA in the community will depend on the local epidemiological situation. If spread of MRSA is suspected in a setting where the prevalence so far has been low, it is reasonable to try to contain MRSA by adopting a 'search and destroy' policy. This implies screening according to the 'ring study' principle, where the MRSA-positive client's contacts are screened for MRSA. If their samples are negative, the investigation is discontinued. If they reveal new cases, their contacts are examined, and so on. All identified MRSA carriers are offered eradication therapy, if possible (see below). These principles have so far been successfully practised in community settings in low-prevalence countries, such as The Netherlands[20] and Denmark.[9,12] In societies where MRSA is more prevalent, this strategy may not be practicable and containment programmes will have to be less ambitious.

Microbiological testing is still largely based on cultures, but new and rapid tests based on the detection of the mecA gene or its products are becoming available. In order to detect or rule out MRSA carriage, it is necessary as a minimum to take swabs from the following three sites: (i) both nostrils (using the same swab); (ii) the throat; and (iii) the perineum.

Swabs should also be taken from open wounds and other skin lesions, if present. Insertion sites of in-dwelling catheters should also be cultured, and a urine culture should be performed from clients with in-dwelling urinary catheters.

With the present laboratory techniques for processing of screening samples, false-negative results occur and it may be necessary to repeat sampling, particularly if the client/patient is on antibiotic treatment.

Nursing homes and other long-term care facilities

Nursing homes and other long-term care facilities give rise to special problems in regards to control of MRSA. These problems have been dealt with in previous guidelines from the British Society for Antimicrobial Chemotherapy and the Hospital Infection Society.[21]

Sharing facilities day after day implies a risk for transmission of MRSA among clients, once the organism has been introduced. Old facilities not designed for containment of contagious agents and staff lacking experience with infection control may further enhance problems. Until now, most MRSA-colonised residents in nursing homes have acquired their MRSA strains during hospitalisation. Experience shows that these strains have little tendency to spread to other residents; however, this situation may change with the introduction of new and more virulent MRSA clones from the community (Table 14.2).

Guidelines for nursing homes and other long-term care facilities are faced with special challenges, because they deal with a setting, which is to be regarded as the client's own home. They have to be effective, but at the same time not too restrictive, in order to remain human and socially acceptable. In the past, there has been much anxiety about the spread of MRSA, and MRSA-positive patients have been denied admission to nursing homes when discharged from hospitals. In general, there is no sound reason for that.

> If simple hygienic precautions are followed, MRSA carriers are not a hazard to relatives, residents, staff or other community members.[21]

In order to cope with MRSA and other infection problems, each residential facility should have an infection control policy and a designated person responsible for infection control matters. Policies and guidelines should be worked out in close liaison with local experts (microbiologist, infection control nurse, medical officer of health), who may also be involved in the training of staff.

The following precautions should be adopted if MRSA has been demonstrated in a client:

1. If possible, the client should have a private room. This is particularly important if the client has open wounds or other conditions, where MRSA can propagate. Married couples can continue sharing rooms.

2. All procedures related to treatment and care should take place in the client's private room.

3. The client is free to take part in social activities outside his/her private room.

4. The client and his/her visitors should be instructed in essential precautions, particularly hand hygiene to be performed before leaving the room.

5. Open wounds should be coated with dry, tight-fitting dressings, which should be changed regularly in order to avoid percolation.

6. Adjuncts related to treatment and care should, if possible, be reserved for use in the MRSA-positive client. If not, they must be decontaminated properly before being used for other clients.

7. Staff engaged in the treatment and care of MRSA-positive clients should be instructed properly in relevant infection control procedures, including hand hygiene and the use of gloves and gowns and other personal protective means.

8. Staff should not wear their private clothes, when treating and caring for MRSA-positive clients.

9. If the client is hospitalised or treated in out-patient facilities, the attending staff should be informed about the client's MRSA status, so that proper containment measures can be taken. Similarly, the nursing-home manager should be informed by the hospital, when a MRSA-positive client is discharged and transferred to a nursing home.

If possible, attempts should be made to eradicate MRSA carriage. If this is not possible, e.g. due to the presence of underlying conditions (see below), consideration should be given to offering the client one or two weekly showers with 4% chlorhexidine liquid soap or povidone iodine shampoo in order to reduce the inoculum of MRSA and, thereby, the risk of transmitting the organism to staff and other clients.

After successful eradication of MRSA carriage in a client or after the client has vacated the room permanently, it should be spring-cleaned. This includes the following elements:

1. Curtains and linen are machine-washed at a minimum of 65°C.[22]

2. Mattress covers are cleaned and wiped with a suitable disinfectant.

3. Mattresses, floors, carpets, cushions and upholstered furniture are vacuum cleaned using a vacuum cleaner with a filter. Bags and filters are changed after vacuum cleaning and disposed of.

4. Pillows, blankets and eiderdowns are washed, if possible at minimum 65°C. It may be necessary to use lower temperatures for heat-labile items. Thorough washing at 40–50°C will remove most organisms and may, if necessary, be supplemented by chemical disinfection.[22]

5. The room is aired.

Clients receiving home care

Home-care staff may run a risk of becoming colonised with MRSA, when caring for a MRSA-positive client. Often, their knowledge about infection control is limited. It is, therefore, essential that they are informed and trained properly, when caring for MRSA positive clients. Most important is to instruct them in hand-washing techniques and, if relevant, they may be provided with bottles of alcoholic hand rub. It is the responsibility of the home-care management to ensure that this takes place. Hospitals discharging MRSA-positive patients to home care should inform the home-care management, so that proper infection control measures can be taken.

When caring for a MRSA-positive client, the following precautions should be taken:

1. Work should be organised so that the fewest possible staff have contact with the client.

2. If possible, the visit to the client's home should be postponed to the end of the working day.

3. Open wounds should be coated with a dry tight-fitting dressing, which should be changed regularly.

4. The client should be instructed in proper hand hygiene before leaving his/her home.

5. Staff engaged in the treatment and care of MRSA-positive clients should be instructed properly in relevant infection control procedures, including hand hygiene and the use of gloves, gowns/plastic aprons and other barrier precautions.

6. Staff should not wear their private clothes, when treating and caring for MRSA-positive clients.

7. If possible, attempts should be made to eradicate MRSA carriage, along the lines given below.

Schools, kindergartens and day-care centres

A good hygienic standard with special emphasis on hand hygiene and domestic cleaning is the most effective way to control MRSA in schools and day-care institutions. Managers must ensure that there is a good provision of hand-washing facilities (basins, liquid soap, and paper towels), and children, clients and staff should be instructed in their proper use.

Children and clients with impetigo and other major skin and wound infections must be kept at home until their lesions have healed. However, there are no restrictions for asymptomatic carriers of MRSA. They are allowed to go to schools and day-care centres, and they can participate in all activities.

Outbreaks should be investigated by the local medical officer of health along the lines given below. In boarding schools, room mates should be looked upon as household members and treated simultaneously with a MRSA-positive individual, irrespective of their MRSA status.

Day-care centres for clients with physical and mental handicaps may have special problems in relation to MRSA, partly because clients have frequent hospital contacts, and partly because

MRSA is easily spread in these settings. If MRSA is demonstrated in a client in such an institution, all clients, or at least those who have contact with the colonised individual, should be offered a MRSA screen; colonised individuals should be offered treatment for their MRSA carriage.

Clinics (medical, dental, physiotherapy, pedicure, etc.)

The general precautions against contact transmission (see above) form the basis for control of MRSA in all types of clinics. If necessary, the clinic should have its procedures examined by an infection control nurse in order to ensure that these precautions are fully understood and implemented. In addition, the following specific precautions should be considered when dealing with a MRSA-colonised individual:

1. A MRSA-positive individual has the same right to treatment as any other citizen. Necessary treatment must not be postponed because of MRSA carriage. On the other hand, if treatment is not urgent, it may be considered prudent to postpone a visit to a clinic till after eradication therapy has been successfully completed.

2. MRSA-positive individuals are encouraged to inform staff in clinics they visit about their MRSA status.

3. If possible, any visit to a clinic should be scheduled to the end of a working day so that proper decontamination and cleaning can be performed before receiving new patients and clients.

4. Stay in the waiting room should be minimised or, if possible, avoided.

Ambulances, taxis and public transport

If a MRSA-positive patient is to be transported in an ambulance, the following precautions should be taken:

1. Chronic wounds must be covered with a tight fitting dressing by the discharging unit.

2. The ambulance staff should be informed that the patient is MRSA positive.

3. The patient should be collected from his/her accommodation and taken directly to the destination, according to instructions given by the ordering unit.

4. If the ambulance staff are in close physical contact with the patient, they should wear gloves and, if necessary, also gowns or aprons for protection of their uniform. Hands should be washed or disinfected with alcohol immediately after the patient has been brought to his/her destination.

5. Sheets and blankets, which have been in direct contact with the patient, should be machine-washed at a minimum of 65°C.

6. Trolleys and other types of equipment that have been in direct contact with the patient should be washed with a detergent or wiped with a disinfectant.

> MRSA-positive clients can use taxies and public transport without any restriction, provided the following measures are taken:

7. Chronic wounds should be covered with a tight fitting dressing.

8. Clients should be dressed in clean clothes.

9. Before transport, they should wash and disinfect their hands.

Treatment of MRSA carriers and follow-up

As a rule, MRSA carriage cannot be eliminated in the presence of wounds and in-dwelling catheters. The same applies to flare-ups of chronic skin disorders (e.g. eczema and psoriasis). These conditions must be controlled before MRSA eradication can be successfully accomplished.

> Treatment of MRSA carriage consists of the following three elements, which are continued for 5 days:

1. Application of mupirocin 2% nasal ointment three times daily to both nostrils.

2. Daily, whole-body showering (including the hair) with 4% chlorhexidine liquid soap or povidone iodine shampoo.

3. Daily changes of clothing, wash cloth, and bath towel, which should be machine-washed at a minimum of 65°C.

During eradication treatment, no other types of soap should be used. In particular, anionic soaps must be avoided, since they reduce the bactericidal effect of chlorhexidine. Body lotions and moisturisers may be used to protect the skin from drying, provided they do not contain anionic compounds.

Household members of a MRSA carrier should be treated simultaneously in order to avoid cross contamination, irrespective of their MRSA status.

> Mupirocin and whole-body wash is not sufficient to eradicate MRSA in throat carriers. In these cases, it is necessary to give a supplementary treatment with systemically administered antibiotics that can reach high concentrations on mucous membranes. Suitable agents include clindamycin or rifampicin combined with fusidic acid, depending on the results of antimicrobial susceptibility testing.

Cleaning the environment is an important part of MRSA eradication. The following should be done after 2 days, and repeated on the last day of treatment:

1. Thorough cleaning of the client's room/home including floor-washing.

2. Vacuum cleaning of carpets, cushions, upholstered furniture, and mattresses, using a vacuum cleaner with filter.

3. Change of bed clothes, which should be machine-washed at a minimum of 65°C.

Pillows, blankets and eiderdowns are washed on the last day of treatment.

The result of eradication treatment is checked by cultures. These are taken 1, 2, and 3 weeks after the termination of treatment. Cultures should, as a minimum, be taken from nostrils and throat and, if necessary, from other sites where MRSA has previously been demonstrated.

In case of treatment failure the following issues should be addressed:

- did the patient comply fully with the regimen?
- are there underlying conditions (see above) that were not controlled sufficiently before eradication therapy was started?
- is the patient a throat carrier?
- is the strain resistant to mupirocin?
- has the environment been cleaned sufficiently?
- were all household members treated simultaneously? – if no, could the patient have become re-colonised from an untreated household member?
- are there pets in the household that could be MRSA carriers?

References

1. Saïd-Salim B, Mathema B, Kreiswirth BN. Community-acquired methicillin-resistant *Staphylococcus aureus*: an emerging pathogen. *Infect Control Hosp Epidemiol* 2003; **24**: 451–5.

2. Weber JT. Community-associated methicillin-resistant Staphylococcus aureus. *Clin Infect Dis* 2005; **41**: S269–72.

3. Salgado CD, Farr BM, Calfee DP. Community-acquired methicillin-resistant *Staphylococcus aureus*: a meta-analysis of prevalence and risk factors. *Clin Infect Dis* 2003; **36**: 131–9.

4. Crossley K. Long-term care facilities as sources of antibiotic-resistant nosocomial pathogens. *Curr Opin Infect Dis* 2001; **14**: 455–9.

5. Borer A, Gilad J, Yagupsky P et al. Community-acquired methicillin-resistant *Staphylococcus aureus* in institutionalized adults with developmental disabilities. *Emerg Infect Dis* 2002; **8**: 966–70.

6. Anon. Methicillin-resistant *Staphylococcus aureus* infections in correctional facilities – Georgia, California, and Texas, 2001–2003. *MMWR* 2003; **52**: 992–6.

7. Zinderman CE, Connor B, Malakooti MA et al. Community-acquired methicillin-resistant *Staphylococcus aureus* among military recruits. *Emerg Infect Dis* 2004; **10**: 941–4.

8. Nguyen DM, Mascola L, Bancroft E. Recurring methicillin-resistant *Staphylococcus aureus* infections in a football team. *Emerg Infect Dis* 2005; **11**: 526–32.

9. Urth T, Juul G, Skov R et al. Spread of methicillin-resistant *Staphylococcus aureus* ST80-IV clone in a Danish community. *Infect Control Hosp Epidemiol* 2005; **26**: 144–9.

10. Sherertz RJ, Bassetti S, Bassetti-Wyss B. 'Cloud' health care workers. *Emerg Infect Dis* 2001; **7**: 241–4.

11. Chambers HF. Community-associated MRSA – resistance and virulence converge. *N Engl J Med* 2005; **352**: 1485–7.

12. Faria NA, Oliveira DC, Westh H et al. Epidemiology of emerging methicillin-resistant *Staphylococcus aureus* (MRSA) in Denmark: a nationwide study in a country with low prevalence of MRSA infection. *J Clin Microbiol* 2005; **43**: 1836–42.

13. Fridkin SK, Hageman JC, Morrison M et al. Methicillin-resistant *Staphylococcus aureus* disease in three communities. *N Engl J Med* 2005; **352**: 1436–44.

14. Miller LG, Perdreau-Remington F, Rieg G et al. Necrotizing fasciitis caused by community-associated methicillin-resistant *Staphylococcus aureus* in Los Angeles. *N Engl J Med* 2005; **352**: 1445–53.

15. Gillet Y, Issartel B, Vanhems P et al. Association between *Staphylococcus aureus* strains carrying gene for Panton-Valentine leukocidin and highly lethal necrotizing pneumonia in young immunocompetent patients. *Lancet* 2002; **359**: 753–9.

16. Kourbatova EV, Halvosa JS, King MD et al. Emergence of community-associated methicillin-resistant *Staphylococcus aureus* USA 300 clone as a cause of health care-associated infections among patients with prosthetic joint infections. *Am J Infect Control* 2005; **33**: 385–91.

17. Saiman L, O'Keefe M, Graham III PL et al. Hospital transmission of community-acquired methicillin-resistant *Staphylococcus aureus* among postpartum women. *Clin Infect Dis* 2003; **37**: 1313–9.

18. Babb J. Decontamination of the environment, equipment and the skin. In: Ayliffe GAJ, Fraise AP, Geddes AM, Mitchell K. (eds) *Control of hospital infection. A practical handbook*. London: Arnold, 2000; 92–128.

19. International Federation of Infection Control (IFIC). *Basic concepts and training,* 2nd edn. <http://www.theific.org>.

20. Dutch Working Party Infection Prevention (WIP). *MRSA in nursing homes*. September 2005. <http://www.wip.nl>.

21. Duckworth G, Heathcock R. Working Party Report. Guidelines on the control of methicillin-resistant Staphylococcus aureus in the community. Report of a combined working party by the British Society for Antimicrobial Chemotherapy and the Hospital Infection Society. *J Hosp Infect* 1995; **31**: 1–12.

22. Barrie D. Laundry hygiene and handling of contaminated linen. In: Ayliffe GAJ, Fraise AP, Geddes AM, Mitchell K. (eds) *Control of hospital infection. A practical handbook*. London: Arnold, 2000; 239–43.

15. The SISS MRSA guidance: risk assessment and targeted screening

Dugald Baird

A Scottish perspective
Background – a steadily increasing pool of colonised patients
The SISS guidance
Principles of the approach

Independently, the Scottish Infection Standards and Strategy Group (SISS) of The Royal College of Physicians of Edinburgh and The Royal College of Physicians and Surgeons of Glasgow convened a sub-group to address the specific issue of MRSA in the hospital setting, considering that it would be helpful to take a fresh look at the problem and suggest new guidance for its control, as current methods as practised in most hospitals are manifestly not working. Figure 15.1 shows the experience of a typical Scottish hospital which was virtually free of MRSA until the arrival of the current 'epidemic' strains in the mid 1990s, since when the numbers of identified patients continued to increase, in spite of valiant efforts by infection control staff in introducing generally accepted conventional good practice measures.

A Scottish perspective

Concern over healthcare-associated infection (HAI) in Scotland resulted in the publication of the Ministerial HAI Action Plan in October 2002 and the establishment of the HAI Task Force, whose work is on-going. Several important documents have already emerged from this exercise, including the *Code of Practice for the Local Management of Hygiene and Healthcare Associated Infection*.

The Scottish Infection Standards and Strategy Group (SISS) of The Royal College of Physicians of Edinburgh and The Royal College of Physicians and Surgeons of Glasgow is a multidisciplinary team of professionals whose work involves coping with infections. Projects to date have included the development of standards for healthcare-associated infection, sexually transmitted infections, *Escherichia coli* 0157 and antimicrobial prescribing.

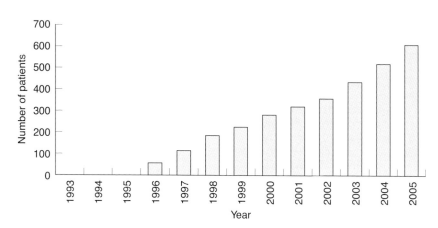

Figure 15.1
Numbers of patients identified with MRSA in a Scottish district general hospital, 1993–2005.

The SISS guidance was published in 2006 as a robust contribution to the MRSA debate. It has one aim: to reduce the incidence of MRSA infections in patients, and is intended to be a 'hands-on' document. It is, therefore, addressed principally to clinical nursing and medical staff, infection control teams and bed managers, although of course hospital administrators have a key role in support and facilitation. This chapter briefly presents some of the available evidence that led to the production of this guidance and contains its key section – 'Management of patients at the time of admission'. The full document also gives suggestions as to the antibiotic treatment of MRSA infections, good laboratory practice, and addresses the sensitive issue of screening healthcare staff for MRSA carriage.

Background – a steadily increasing pool of colonised patients

MRSA has now been endemic in most UK hospitals for at least a decade (Fig. 15.1), and this has allowed a significant build up of carriers in the population here as elsewhere, due to the exportation of 'hospital' strains and subsequent transmission to family or care home contacts of discharged patients. In 1994, Fraise *et al.* found that 17% of residents of a Birmingham nursing home were MRSA carriers. (The role of the newer true 'community' strains, not associated with admission to hospital, is not yet defined, but is certainly small at present in the UK).

With an ageing population making ever increasing demands on the healthcare system, it is inevitable that the number of patients bringing MRSA into hospital with them will increase, although the scale of this problem certainly differs widely between different populations, clinical units, and types of hospital. In the same hospital as in Figure 15.1, the proportion of all patients discovered to be MRSA carriers who were already known from previous admissions rose from a half to two-thirds between 2003 and 2005.

Many accounts of how MRSA was 'controlled' in a variety of endemic and outbreak situations have been published during the past quarter century and it is clear that there are many ways to do effective infection control. However, no clear consensus emerges as to which practice or practices are of most value in preventing transmission of MRSA in hospitals, and indeed most infection control specialists would agree that it is packages of measures that work most effectively. Unfortunately, the contents of the packages vary considerably. Marshall and colleagues provide a useful critical review of the difficulties involved in disentangling the effects of the variables.

Active searching for MRSA carriers

Against this background of uncertainty, evidence is steadily emerging for the role of active searching for MRSA carriers as a crucial component of control. Many reportedly successful programmes have been based on early identification of patients colonised with MRSA and prompt implementation of contact precautions for them, rather than standard precautions. This has applied both in the control of outbreaks and also in the endemic situation faced by many hospitals in the UK and world-wide.

As long ago as 1982, Thompson *et al.* found that a third of their patients with MRSA were detected only by active screening, but it is only more recently that this issue has again become widely addressed. A flurry of recent publications has demonstrated that only a proportion, often small, of the total pool of MRSA is uncovered by relying on its isolation from specimens taken for clinical purposes. In other words, infected patients represent 'the tip of the iceberg'.

The 'iceberg' phenomenon

All the best infection control practice in the world will not succeed unless we know who the carriers are, and this is the central message of the SISS document. This is supported by a growing body of evidence from around the world.

Who should be screened? – clinical risk assessment

Screening patients for MRSA on admission cannot by itself guide initial patient placement and management, since using conventional methods the laboratory diagnosis of MRSA in a specimen takes a minimum of 24 hours (and usually 48–72 hours). All patients need, therefore, to be clinically assessed on admission to hospital, so that those with risk factors for MRSA can be managed with contact precautions right from the beginning. Management can subsequently be modified if necessary, depending on laboratory confirmation or otherwise of their MRSA status. It is in this greater emphasis on clinical assessment of all admissions that the SISS guidance mainly differs from the recently revised UK Joint Working Party guidelines and the Irish guidelines.

> *Clinical risk assessment*
>
> This is simply finding the answers to a few key questions, since we know that certain categories of patients are more likely to be MRSA carriers. The guidance advises that any patient who falls into one or more of these categories is automatically regarded as a suspect MRSA carrier and is treated as such pending laboratory confirmation or otherwise.

MRSA is, of course, not the only pathogen of concern in health-associated infection, and some hospitals have adopted a risk assessment for infection of all types, performed as part of the routine admission documentation, which is intended to identify which patients may harbour potentially transmissible pathogens. Specific enquiry for generally accepted MRSA risk factors can easily be incorporated into such an assessment; a suggested example of how this could be done, based on an NHS Greater Glasgow protocol, can be found in the full SISS guidance which is available from the website of The Royal College of Physicians of Edinburgh.

Targeted screening

Patients who should undergo microbiological screening to determine whether or not they do carry MRSA are those identified by this clinical risk assessment as more likely MRSA carriers. This targeted screening need not be unduly onerous and, to be practicable, the number of samples taken should be as few as possible. Nasal swabs alone will detect between 75–97% of carriers, while sensitivity is increased if additional swabs are taken from breaks in the skin and a sample of urine obtained from catheterised patients. The task of form filling is simplified by the use of preprinted laboratory forms which only require boxes to be ticked and a patient identification label applied.

> *Targeted screening*
>
> This is the taking of one or a few swabs for microbiological identification from those patients whose clinical risk assessment suggests are at higher risk of being MRSA carriers. Laboratory methods need to be as quick as possible compatible with accuracy, and technical methods are rapidly changing to meet this demand.

The size of the 'silent' MRSA pool

Many studies have now investigated the size of the imported pool of MRSA carriers in a variety of clinical settings, using either universal or targeting screening (based on various combinations of risk factors). Authors have had differing views on whether targeted screening is sufficiently sensitive to detect most carriers. For example, Girou et al. compared the results of targeted screening with universal screening of patients admitted to a dermatology ward, and found no difference in the prevalence of MRSA, suggesting that the criteria adopted for screening were well judged. Targeted screening was, however, much more cost-effective. On the other hand, Lucet et al. found that only universal screening was acceptably sensitive in an ICU. The SISS group adopted the majority view that targeted screening should be the recommended procedure, on grounds of proven efficacy and cost-effectiveness. However, some hospitals are already screening all admissions to selected units and, if this is proving beneficial, then of course it should continue.

How big is the MRSA pool?

This depends on the patient population, the criteria used for screening, and the type of clinical unit. However, the rapidly mounting evidence from around the world suggests that about 5% of all hospital admissions carry MRSA, higher in elderly populations and in some specialised units. In a rare UK study, Samad and colleagues found a prevalence of 5.3% MRSA carriers amongst admissions to surgical wards of a Welsh hospital.

In most reports, without active screening, MRSA would have been undetected in at least half of newly admitted patients. Specimens sent to the microbiology laboratory for clinical reasons only detect a proportion (often small) of all the patients with MRSA, so that in many, if not most, acute clinical units in the UK and elsewhere, many patients carrying MRSA are not managed with appropriate infection control nursing precautions – a recent US study showed that screening cultures were performed in only 30% of healthcare facilities.

Why hunt for asymptomatic carriers, and how should they be managed?

The main purpose of actively identifying known or suspected MRSA carriers on admission is so that appropriate infection control measures can be applied to all patients as soon as possible. In addition, as carriage is a risk factor for subsequent infection, patients may also benefit from pro-active clinical management (see chapters by Seaton and Nathwani).

Antibiotic-resistant strains of *Staphylococcus aureus* seem always to have shown increased transmissibility in patients receiving antibiotics, and the propensity for spread of contemporary strains of MRSA is everyday

hospital experience. The much quoted study by Jernigan *et al.* showed that transmission of MRSA from colonised or infected patients was some 15-fold less when these patients were nursed in isolation with contact precautions than when in open wards using standard precautions. This advantage was only slightly reduced when the data were later re-worked to include only colonised patients, omitting those with overt infections. The fact that these studies involved neonates who stay where they are put, which represents a very different situation from adults who tend to move about, contaminating their immediate environment, only strengthens the evidence. The Jernigan study is important because it is one of the few attempting to quantify the benefit of contact precautions.

Isolation of known or suspected carriers

The role of patient isolation has been questioned, but not convincingly; therefore, the SISS guidance advises isolation, or at least cohorting, wherever possible for known or suspected carriers. It is of course recognised that, in some situations, sheer numbers of patients and antiquated ward design make this well-nigh impossible. In these circumstances, priority for single-room accommodation should be given to those patients perceived as posing the greatest risk of dissemination of MRSA, for example those who have MRSA on the skin as well as in the nose, or who are catheterised. Individual patient factors should, however, also be taken into account. The views of Bissett and Makoni are helpful in this respect. Humphreys draws attention to the fact that: 'where bed occupancy rates are high, it is unlikely that there will be the flexibility within the system to facilitate adequate isolation and cohorting of patients during outbreaks'. Nevertheless, an attempt should always be made and, where isolation facilities are unavailable or inappropriate for particular patients, those with MRSA and those without MRSA, should be kept apart as far as is possible.

Should all MRSA carriers and suspected carriers be isolated?

Probably yes, since they are then much less likely to be active reservoirs for transmission. The decision to isolate must remain a clinical one, but a change of patients' and visitors' attitudes to isolation would not be impossible if a national MRSA infection-reduction strategy became policy.

Would the proposals work?

Would the wide-spread adoption of clinical risk assessment and targeted screening as a guide to patient management reduce the number of healthcare-associated MRSA infections, and would this be cost-effective?

Common sense suggests that reducing cross-infection would automatically reduce the number of cases of infection by hospital-acquired MRSA, though hard evidence for this is found in only a relatively few reports. Girou *et al.* screened admissions to a medical ICU with MRSA risk factors and nursed identified patients in isolation. During the study period the prevalence of imported cases did not change but the incidence of ICU-acquired cases fell from 5.6% to 1.4%. In a similar study, Boyce *et al.* reduced the proportion of patients who developed MRSA infections in their ICU from 2.2% to 0.7%.

Wernitz *et al.* estimated that a selective admission screening programme over 19 months prevented nearly half of the predicted number of acquired MRSA infections, at a saving of over 100,000 euros per year. The programme was calculated to be cost efficient at even a low prevalence of MRSA in admissions.

In a case-controlled study, Chaix demonstrated a 14% fall in MRSA infection rates in an ICU when patients found to have MRSA by screening were isolated and managed with contact precautions, compared with those who had not been screened and subsequently acquired MRSA in the unit. The mean cost of treating patients who acquired MRSA was $9275, whereas the

screening and intervention programme cost $340–1480 per patient.

West *et al.*, employing targeted screening and isolation of colonised patients, reduced the rate of nosocomial MRSA infections, and saved money.

Would the guidance work?

Studies world-wide are appearing with increasing frequency. It seems that looking for MRSA and managing it does work. The question is becoming not 'how' but 'when' do we start to take action: 'It is time to take action, make patient safety a priority, and put the fire out' (Muto).

The SISS guidance

What follows is a summary of the suggested approach to MRSA control prepared by the SISS MRSA subgroup. Active surveillance for MRSA carriers lies at the core of the guidelines issued in 2003 by the Society of Healthcare Epidemiology of America. The SISS group also unequivocally recommended this approach as the mainstay of a package of control measures.

The guidance itself is simple in principle, though difficult in practice. It complements and does not replace existing best infection control practice. It cannot be too strongly emphasised that it is very unlikely that this or any other any attempts at MRSA control would work unless a robust and high quality infection control infrastructure were in place, with adequate resources, both human and environmental, as essential components. Without these, any attempts to control healthcare-associated infections are bound to fail. Worse, the measures proposed could simply add meaningless extra burdens on to the shoulders of already hard-pressed clinical, infection control and laboratory staff.

Principles of the approach

1. A documented clinical risk assessment of all newly admitted patients must be done

to identify patients for whom infection with MRSA could be especially dangerous, and also those who are more likely to be carriers of MRSA. A patient can of course belong to both categories.

2. This clinical risk assessment must be supplemented by targeted surveillance for MRSA.

3. Patient care management must conform to existing best practice infection control guidance.

4. Carriage of MRSA by healthcare workers must be considered in certain epidemic situations, such as failure to control outbreaks, or the unexplained appearance in a clinical area of new or especially pathogenic strains of MRSA. Such carriage by staff may be transient or longer term, and has probably not always received the attention it deserves.

5. Each healthcare institution must review its antimicrobial formulary and prescribing practices policy and amend them if necessary in line with best practice guidance.

6. Cleaning of healthcare environments and equipment must conform to existing best practice guidance.

7. The microbiology laboratory identification of MRSA in a specimen must be as rapid as possible, given the absolute requirement for accuracy.

The term 'high risk' was avoided because of the ambiguity that sometimes arises between whether one is referring to patients at risk, or posing a risk. The terms used, 'vulnerable patients', 'unlikely MRSA carriers' and 'possible MRSA carriers' are not ideal, but unambiguously convey the meanings intended.

Implementation of the guidance

Some hospitals are already using essentially the same approach as recommended, at least in some clinical units. Hospitals should ultimately aim to implement this guidance for all patients. Clearly, this is for many not an immediate possibility. A distinction is, therefore, made

between 'acute clinical units' and 'non-acute clinical units', which is simply intended to distinguish between clinical units where invasive procedures of all types are routinely performed, and those where such procedures are less common. Clearly the distinction is not absolute, and each hospital must decide on its own categorisation.

Management of patients at the time of admission

Aim

To identify as quickly as possible which newly admitted patients are: (i) vulnerable to MRSA infection; (ii) especially vulnerable; (iii) possible MRSA carriers; and (iv) unlikely MRSA carriers. These groups should then be nursed as far apart as possible.

Definitions

A list of definitions used in the SISS guidance is given in Table 15.1.

Clinical risk assessment

All patients should undergo a clinical risk assessment for possible infection, including MRSA, as part of the routine admission process (unless already done at a recent pre-admission assessment clinic). In most cases, the risk assessment can be performed by a simple questionnaire or perusal of the patient case record. A suggested proforma is available from the website of The Royal College of Physicians of Edinburgh within the full SISS guidance, and a few illustrative examples are given in Appendix II.

Targeted surveillance (selective screening for MRSA)

Patients admitted to acute clinical units whose risk assessment suggests they are 'possible MRSA carriers' should be screened for MRSA (targeted surveillance). Targeted surveillance for MRSA should also be done in 'non-acute clinical areas' if the clinical risk assessment and/or local factors dictate, e.g. the presence

Table 15.1
A list of definitions used in the SISS guidance

Acute clinical unit	A clinical area where patients are at increased risk of infection with MRSA because of invasive procedures, wounds or skin/soft tissue lesions
Non-acute clinical unit	A clinical area where the above do not apply. Examples might be long-stay care of the elderly units, psychiatric units, *etc.*, but local categorisation of units is required
Clinical risk assessment	Assessment of a patient as 'vulnerable', 'especially vulnerable', 'unlikely MRSA carrier' or 'possible MRSA carrier' by questioning the patient/relative and/or perusal of the case record. It should form part of the general admission assessment for infection. In the case of elective admissions, these procedures could have been performed prior to admission, at pre-admission assessment.
Vulnerable patient	A patient admitted to an acute clinical unit; also patients in non-acute units who have significant organic medical or surgical conditions
Especially vulnerable patient	A patient who is to undergo surgery to implant foreign material of any type
Possible MRSA carrier	A patient with one or more risk factors for MRSA carriage identified by clinical risk assessment
Unlikely MRSA carrier	A patient with no risk factors for MRSA carriage identified by clinical risk assessment
Targeted surveillance	Microbiological screening of patients identified as possible MRSA carriers to find out if they do in fact carry MRSA
Isolation	Placing a patient in a single room and using appropriate infection control precautions either to prevent spread of MRSA from the patient or to prevent the patient acquiring MRSA, as appropriate
Cohorting	Placing a patient in a designated area of the ward together with other similar patients, *i.e.* either known/suspected to be carrying MRSA or known to be free of MRSA, as appropriate
Topical clearance regimen	A course of nasal ointment plus skin antiseptic given to a patient in order to attempt to remove MRSA carriage

of vulnerable patients in the ward, or if local policy is to attempt eradication/exclusion of MRSA from these clinical areas.

Risk factors for MRSA carriage

Patients who are 'possible MRSA carriers' are those who:

- are known to be carrying MRSA, or to have done so previously
- are admitted from care homes
- have been in hospital within the past 12 months
- are transferred from other hospitals or from abroad

- have received repeated course of antibiotics
- have renal disease or diabetes
- have skin breaks (*e.g.* pressure sores, leg ulcers, intravenous line sites, PEG tubes)
- have certain active dermatological conditions (*e.g.* psoriasis or eczema).

Nursing management

Patients with known or possible MRSA must be nursed away from those without MRSA as much as facilities allow. The clinical risk assessment will help to guide appropriate nursing management (*e.g.* the use of isolation rooms or cohorting, transmission-based precautions) right from the beginning of the patient's admission. In addition, it is good practice to nurse especially vulnerable patients who are unlikely MRSA carriers away from possible MRSA carriers, and isolation should be considered for them if there are known or suspected carriers on the ward.

When the results of the screening for MRSA are known, it may then be possible to modify individual management in order to make best use of scarce resources such as isolation facilities. If pre-admission screening for MRSA has been done and the results are known at the time of admission, optimum use of these facilities can be made immediately.

Single rooms are generally a scarce resource; when isolation facilities are unavailable or inappropriate, patients with and without MRSA should wherever possible be cohorted separately. Suggestions for priority for isolation rooms are given below.

Summary of management

This is summarised in the following and in the flow chart in Appendix I. Some illustrative examples are given in Appendix II.

Newly admitted patients

Patients who are already known to be MRSA carriers should be isolated (cohorted), a full MRSA screen performed, and started on a topical clearance regimen unless this is contra-indicated.

Patients whose MRSA status is unknown but who are regarded as possible carriers (by the above criteria) should be isolated (cohorted) and an admission screen performed. When the result of this screen is known, patients who are negative can usually be nursed in the open ward. Patients found to be positive should continue to be isolated, have a full MRSA screen performed, and be commenced on a topical clearance regimen unless this is contra-indicated. When non-isolated patients are found to be positive, their contacts should then be screened.

Patients who are regarded as unlikely carriers by these criteria and also those known to be recently negative can be nursed in the open ward and need not be screened, although consideration should be given to screening and isolating especially vulnerable patients in these groups, for example if there are known MRSA carriers in the same clinical unit.

Subsequent management

It is usual to advise that patients who have undergone one or more courses of MRSA clearance treatment remain in isolation until three consecutive negative full screens at intervals of not less than 48 hours have been obtained. Vulnerable patients should be re-screened (nose, skin breaks) weekly if there are patients in the same clinical area with MRSA. Patients moved from a non-acute to an acute clinical area should undergo the MRSA screen if not already performed.

Isolation

Isolation facilities are usually limited. Priority should, therefore, be given to two distinct categories of patients:

1. Especially vulnerable patients who are unlikely MRSA carriers, if there are patients with MRSA in the same clinical area.

2. Patients who are more likely to be shedders of MRSA, *i.e.* who have MRSA on the skin as well as in the nose, or who are catheterised.

When isolation facilities are unavailable or inappropriate for particular patients, those with MRSA and those without MRSA should, wherever possible, be cohorted separately.

Practical aspects of screening for MRSA
Initial screen

Nasal swabs are taken in all cases. A single swab should be used, inserted into both anterior nares in turn to a depth of 1 cm and gently rotated, then placed into the transport medium, labelled and bagged immediately, and sent without delay to the microbiology laboratory. In addition, swabs should be taken from any areas of broken skin, and a specimen of urine taken from catheterised patients. Request forms should indicate that they are for MRSA screening, and the microbiology laboratory should 'fast-track' these specimens.

Full screen

Further swabs should be taken from patients who are positive on initial screening, *i.e.* throat, perineum, any skin breaks, and urine if catheterised. Following a course of clearance therapy, a further full screen should be done as above. Three consecutive negative screens taken at intervals of not less than 48 hours are usually accepted for practical purposes as successful clearance, at least in the short-term.

Clearance of MRSA carriage

This should normally be attempted in all patients carrying MRSA who are in acute clinical units.

Contact patients

Contact patients are defined here as in-patients who have been cared for in close proximity to the positive patient ('index case'), *i.e.* in adjacent beds, or in the same 4-bedded room, for example, for a minimum of 12 hours. (There are no data on the minimum time that contacts have to share the same environment to have a high risk of acquiring MRSA, but it is suggested that a minimum of 12 hours is realistic. This may need to be modified in the light of local experience, and may differ in different clinical settings). Contact patients who are screened and found positive are then managed as for index cases.

Screening of staff

Screening of staff whose work involves close physical contact with patients (*e.g.* nurses, doctors, physiotherapists) for MRSA carriage should be considered when an unexplained persistent increase in the number of patients with MRSA occurs in an acute clinical unit or when new or especially pathogenic strains appear.

Appendix I

Initial management of patients on admission to acute clinical unit

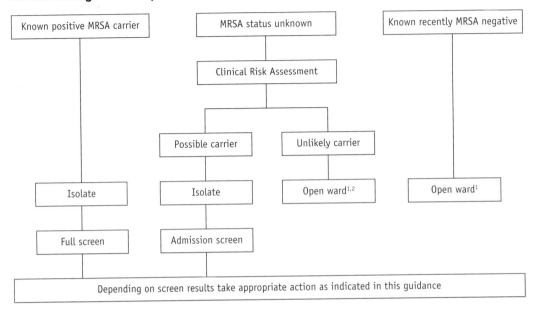

[1] Consider isolation for own protection if especially vulnerable
[2] Consider screening if especially vulnerable

Appendix II

Examples of initial management

1. A patient in good general health is admitted at 10 am from home for elective joint replacement surgery. She had attended pre-admission assessment, was screened for MRSA, and found to be negative.

Clinical risk assessment put the patient into the 'especially vulnerable' category and, therefore, nursing staff have precise information on which to plan management. A single room is available, and isolation is indicated because the staff know that there is/are one or more patients in the ward with MRSA.

2. A patient with a chronic medical condition and many previous admissions is admitted as an emergency at 9 pm to an acute medical receiving ward. Many patients admitted at the same time have similar medical histories. There is no recent information on MRSA status, and single rooms are unavailable.

Clinical risk assessment puts the patient into the 'possible MRSA carrier' category. Nursing staff will attempt to cohort nurse the patient in an area of the ward with similar patients, and are aware of the importance of meticulous attention to strict infection control precautions to prevent transmission of MRSA to other patients, if the patient is in fact a carrier. Screening swabs will be taken and sent immediately to the microbiology laboratory.

3. An elderly lady from a care home is admitted through accident and emergency having fallen and suffered a fractured neck of femur at 10 pm.

Clinical risk assessment puts the patient into both the 'vulnerable patient' and 'possible MRSA carrier' categories. Nursing staff will, therefore, isolate or at least cohort the patient. Strict observance of infection control precautions is essential to prevent either acquisition of MRSA if she is free of MRSA, or transmission of MRSA to other patients, if the patient is in fact a carrier. Screening swabs will be taken and sent immediately to the microbiology laboratory.

Further reading

Policies

Coia JE, Duckworth G, Edwards DI et al. Guidelines for the Control and Prevention of meticillin-resistant Staphylococcus aureus (MRSA) in healthcare facilities by the joint British Society for Antimicrobial Chemotherapy, Hospital Infection Society and Infection Control Nurses Association Working Party on MRSA. J Hosp Infect 2006; 63 (suppl 1): S1–S44.

Healthcare Associated Infection Task Force. The NHS Scotland Code of Practice for the Local Management of Hygiene and Healthcare Associated Infection. Scottish Executive Edinburgh 2004.

Infection Control Subcommittee, Strategy for the Control of Antimicrobial Resistance in Ireland. The Control and Prevention of MRSA in Hospitals and in the Community. Health Service Executive, Health Protection Surveillance Centre 2005.

Muto CA, Jernigan JA, Ostrowsky BE et al. SHEA guidelines for preventing nosocomial transmission of multidrug-resistant strains of Staphylococcus aureus and Enterococcus. Infect Control Hosp Epidemiol 2003; 24: 362–6.

Preventing infections acquired while receiving healthcare. The Scottish Executive's Action Plan to reduce risk to patients, staff and visitors. Scottish Executive October 2002.

Scottish Infection Standards and Strategy Group. Guidance for the Hospital Management of meticillin-resistant Staphylococcus aureus. Royal College of Physicians and Surgeons of Glasgow and Royal College of Physicians of Edinburgh, March 2006.

Community MRSA

Fraise AP, Mitchell K, O'Brien SJ, Oldfield K, Wise R. Methicillin resistant Staphylococcus aureus (MRSA) in nursing homes in a major UK city: an anonymised point prevalence survey. Epidemiol Infect 1997; 118: 1–5.

Hicks NR, Moore EP, Williams EW. Carriage and community treatment of methicillin-resistant Staphylococcus aureus: what happens to colonised patients after discharge? J Hosp Infect 1991; 19: 17–24.

Salgado CD, Farr BM, Calfee DP. Community-acquired methicillin-resistant Staphylococcus aureus: a meta-analysis of prevalence and risk factors. Clin Infect Dis 2003; 36: 131–9.

Review of MRSA policies

Marshall C, Wesselingh S, McDonald M, Spelman D. Control of endemic MRSA – what is the evidence? A personal view. J Hosp Infect 2004; 56: 253–68.

Voss A. Preventing the spread of MRSA. BMJ 2004; 329: 521.

Active surveillance

Coello R, Jimenez J, Garcia M et al. Prospective study of infection, colonisation and carriage of methicillin-resistant Staphylococcus aureus in an outbreak affecting 900 patients. Eur J Clin Microbiol Infect Dis 1994; 13: 74–81.

Eveillard M, Lancien E, Barnaud G et al. Impact of screening for MRSA carriers at hospital admission on risk-adjusted indicators according to the imported MRSA colonisation pressure. J Hosp Infect 2005; 59: 254–8.

Farr BM, Salgado CD, Karchmer TB, Sherertz RJ. Can antibiotic resistant nosocomial infections be controlled? Lancet Infect Dis 2001; 1: 38–45.

Girou E, Pujade G, Legrand P, Cizeau F, Brun-Buisson C. Selective screening of carriers for control of methicillin-resistant Staphylococcus aureus (MRSA) in high-risk hospital areas with a high level of endemic MRSA. Clin Infect Dis 1998; 27: 543–50.

Gould IM. The clinical significance of methicillin-resistant Staphylococcus aureus. J Hosp Infect 2005; 61: 277–82.

Hori S. Meticillin-resistant Staphylococcus aureus (Japan). Forum. Lancet Infect Dis 2005; 5: 653–63.

Jernigan JA, Pullen AL, Flowers L, Bell M, Jarvis WR. Prevalence of and risk factors for colonisation with methicillin-resistant Staphylococcus aureus at the time of hospital admission. Infect Control Hosp Epidemiol 2003; 24: 409–14.

Jernigan JA, Pullen AL, Partin C, Jarvis WR. Prevalence of and risk factors for colonisation with methicillin-resistant Staphylococcus aureus in an outpatient clinic population. Infect Control Hosp Epidemiol 2003; 24: 445–50.

Lucet JC, Chevret S, Durand-Zaleski I, Chastang C, Regnier B. Prevalence and risk factors for carriage of methicillin-resistant Staphylococcus aureus at admission to the intensive care unit: results of a multicenter study. Arch Intern Med 2003; 163: 181–8.

Lucet JC, Grenet K, Armand-Lefevre L et al. High prevalence of carriage of methicillin-resistant Staphylococcus aureus at hospital admission in elderly patients: implications for infection control strategies. Infect Control Hosp Epidemiol 2005; 26: 121–6.

Manion FA, Senkel D, Zack J, Meyer L. Routine screening for methicillin-resistant Staphylococcus aureus among patients admitted to an acute rehabilitation unit. Infect Control Hosp Epidemiol 2002; 23: 516–19.

Merrer J, Santoli F, Appere-De Vecchi C, Tran B, De Jonghe B, Outin H. 'Colonisation pressure' and risk of acquisition of methicillin-resistant Staphylococcus aureus in a medical intensive care unit. *Infect Control Hosp Epidemiol* 2000; **21**: 718–23.

Papia G, Louie M, Tralla A, Johnson C, Collins V, Simor AE. Screening high-risk patients for methicillin-resistant *Staphylococcus aureus* on admission to the hospital: is it cost effective? *Infect Control Hosp Epidemiol* 1999; **20**: 473–7.

Rubinovitch B, Pittet D. Screening for methicillin-resistant *Staphylococcus aureus* in the endemic hospital: what have we learned? *J Hosp Infect* 2001; **47**: 9–18.

Salgado CD, Nobles DL, Ruisz MS *et al*. Control of nosocomial MRSA with active surveillance cultures and contact precautions. Abstract 28 61 SHEA meeting 2003.

Samad A, Banerjee D, Carbarns N, Ghosh S. Prevalence of methicillin-resistant *Staphylococcus aureus* colonisation in surgical patients on admission to a Welsh hospital. *J Hosp Infect* 2002; **51**: 43–6.

Sunenshine RH, Liedtke LA, Fridkin SK, Strausbaugh LJ, Infectious Diseases Society of America Emerging Infections Network. Management of inpatients colonised or infected with antimicrobial-resistant bacteria in hospitals in the United States. *Infect Control Hosp Epidemiol* 2005; **26**: 138–43.

Talon DR, Bertrand X. Methicillin-resistant *Staphylococcus aureus* in geriatric patients: usefulness of screening in a chronic-care setting. *Infect Control Hosp Epidemiol* 2001; **22**: 505–9.

Thompson RL, Cabezudo I, Wenzel RP. Epidemiology of nosocomial infections caused by methicillin-resistant *Staphylococcus aureus*. *Ann Intern Med* 1982; **97**: 309–17.

Troillet N, Carmeli Y, Samore MH *et al*. Carriage of methicillin-resistant *Staphylococcus aureus* at hospital admission. *Infect Control Hosp Epidemiol* 1998; **19**: 181–5.

Screening

Dancer SJ, Noble WC. Nasal, axillary, and perineal carriage of *Staphylococcus aureus* among women: identification of strains producing epidermolytic toxin. *J Clin Pathol* 1991; **44**: 681–4.

Singh K, Gavin P, Vescio T *et al*. Microbiologic surveillance using nasal cultures alone is sufficient for detection of methicillin-resistant *Staphylococcus aureus* isolates in neonates. *J Clin Microbiol* 2003; **41**: 2755–7.

Transmission of MRSA

Berntsen CA, McDermott W. Increased transmissibility of staphylococci to patients receiving an antimicrobial drug. *N Engl J Med* 1960; **262**: 637–42.

Boyce JM, Potter-Bynoe G, Chenevert C, King T. Environmental contamination due to methicillin-resistant *Staphylococcus aureus*: possible infection control implications. *Infect Control Hosp Epidemiol* 1997; **18**: 622–7.

Geffers C, Farr BM. Risk of transmission of nosocomial methicillin-resistant *Staphylococcus aureus* (MRSA) from patients colonised with MRSA. *Infect Control Hosp Epidemiol* 2005; **26**: 114–5.

Jernigan JA, Titus MG, Groschel DH, Getchell-White SI, Farr BM. Effectiveness of contact isolation during a hospital outbreak of methicillin-resistant *Staphylococcus aureus*. *Am J Epidemiol* 1996; **143**: 496–504.

Vriens MR, Fluit AC, Troelstra A, Verhoef J, van der Werken C. Is methicillin-resistant *Staphylococcus aureus* more contagious than methicillin-susceptible *S. aureus* in a surgical intensive care unit? *Infect Control Hosp Epidemiol* 2002; **23**: 491–4.

Isolation of patients

Beovic B, Bufon T, Cizman M, Kilman J, Skerl M. Isolation of patients with MRSA infection. *Lancet* 2005; **365**: 1304.

Bissett L. Controlling the risk of MRSA infection: screening and isolating patients. *Br J Nurs* 2005; **14**: 386–90.

Cepedia JA, Whitehouse T, Cooper B *et al*. Isolation of patients in single rooms or cohorts to reduce spread of MRSA in intensive-care units: prospective two centre study. *Lancet* 2005; **365**: 295–304.

Cooper BS, Stone SP, Kibbler CC *et al*. Isolation measures in the hospital management of methicillin-resistant *Staphylococcus aureus* (MRSA): systematic review of the literature. *BMJ* 2004; **329**: 533–9.

Humphreys H. Implementing guidelines for the control and prevention of methicillin-resistant *Staphylococcus aureus* and vancomycin-resistant enterococci: how valid are international comparisons of success? *J Hosp Infect* 2006; **62**: 133–5.

Makoni T. MRSA: risk assessment and flexible management. *Nurs Standard* 2002; **16**: 39–41.

Effectiveness

Boyce JM, Havill NL, Kohan C, Dumigan DG, Ligi CE. Do infection control measures work for methicillin-resistant *Staphylococcus aureus*? *Infect Control Hosp Epidemiol* 2004; **25**: 395–401.

Chaix C, Durand-Zaleski I, Alberti C, Brun-Buisson C. Control of epidemic methicillin-resistant *Staphylococcus aureus*: a cost-benefit analysis in an intensive care unit. *JAMA* 1999; **282**: 1745–51.

Health Protection Scotland. Reports on meticillin-resistant *Staphylococcus aureus* bacteraemia in Scotland. <http://www.show.scot.nhs.uk/scieh>.

Jernigan JA, Clemence MA, Stott GA *et al*. Control of methicillin-resistant *Staphylococcus aureus* at a university hospital: one decade later. *Infect Control Hosp Epidemiol* 1995; **16**: 686–96.

Muto CA. Methicillin-resistant *Staphylococcus aureus* control: we didn't start the fire, but it's time to put it out. *Infect Control Hosp Epidemiol* 2003; **27**: 111–5.

Wernitz MH, Swidsinski S, Weist K *et al*. Effectiveness of a hospital-wide selective screening programme for methicillin-resistant *Staphylococcus aureus* (MRSA) carriers at hospital admission to prevent hospital-acquired MRSA infections. *Clin Microbiol Infect* 2005; **11**: 457–65.

Wernitz MH, Keck S, Swidsinski S, Schulz S, Veit SK. Cost analysis of a hospital-wide selective screening programme for methicillin-resistant *Staphylococcus aureus* (MRSA) carriers in the context of diagnosis related groups (DRG) payment. *Clin Microbiol Infect* 2005; **11**: 466–71.

West TE, Guerry C, Hiott M, Morrow M, Ward K, Salgado CD. Effect of targeted surveillance for control of methicillin-resistant *Staphylococcus aureus* in a community hospital system. *Infect Control Hosp Epidemiol* 2006; **27**: 233–8.

16. Surveillance of MRSA

Georgia J Duckworth

Background and definition
What does surveillance do?
Sources of data
Objectives, definitions and dataset
Quality of the data
Numerators, denominators and analysis of the data
Recording and monitoring infections
Feeding back the data and action
Resourcing the surveillance
Conclusions

The prevention and control of methicillin-resistant *Staphylococcus aureus* (MRSA) infections are extremely high profile in the UK. This resulted from surveillance data showing an

inexorable rise in infections throughout the 1990s (Fig. 16.1) and unenviable international comparisons (Fig. 16.2),[1] which then featured in influential reports.[2,3] Surveillance is fundamental to impacting on these high figures, as has been shown by the focus on mandatory surveillance and the setting of targets to drive down current high rates of bacteraemia. This is at its most extreme in England, where trusts with more than 12 MRSA bacteraemias a year are required to meet a 60% reduction target by 2008.[4] Individual trust trajectories have been set, with a minimum 20% reduction per year before 2008. Trust data are published every 6 months, showing numbers and rates by named individual trust.[5] Trust progress is being closely monitored by the Department of Health, the whole system being supervised by the Prime Minister's Delivery Unit. Although this is the extreme end of the spectrum, there are similar schemes operating in other parts of the UK, the collection of MRSA bacteraemia data usually being mandatory, although not always published by a named trust.[6,7] The focus in recent years has been very much on unacceptably high rates of MRSA bacteraemia infection, to the detriment of methicillin-sensitive *S. aureus* (MSSA) surveillance, which has suffered relative

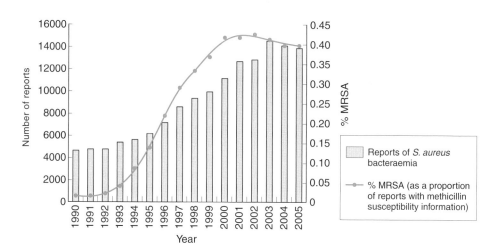

Figure 16.1
S. aureus bacteraemias, England 1990–2005 (source HPA).

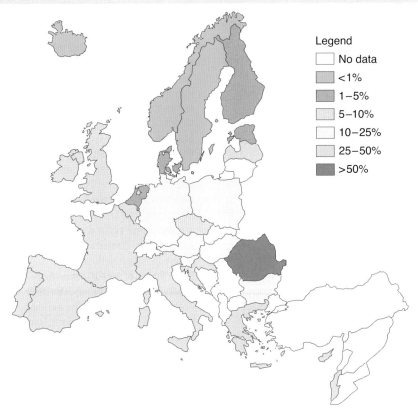

Figure 16.2
S. aureus bacteraemias: proportion resistant to methicillin in 2004 in participating countries (source EARSS).

neglect. MSSA is as important a cause of healthcare-associated infection (HCAI) and surveillance should also encompass MSSA infections to assess whether measures to control MRSA are having an impact on MSSA infections.

Background and definition

The mandatory approach to MRSA surveillance demonstrates that active surveillance is fundamental to the prevention and control of HCAI; control policies are unlikely to be successful in the absence of a planned surveillance programme. Both Semmelweis and Florence Nightingale used surveillance to address widespread infection problems, whilst the SENIC study in the 1970s demonstrated unequivocally

that surveillance is a key component of an infection control programme.[8] Surveillance puts detection of infection on a more solid foundation than indiscriminate, often haphazard, clinical observations on the occurrence of infection. The definition of surveillance as 'information for action' has become hackneyed with use, but is concise. Surveillance is not an end in itself – its role is to measure infection, so that action can be taken to deal with rising or unacceptably high levels.

Surveillance

Information for action to improve the quality of patient care.

A longer, widely accepted, definition which highlights the important components of surveillance is: 'Epidemiologic surveillance is the ongoing systematic collection, analysis, and interpretation of health data essential to the planning, implementation, and evaluation of public health practice, closely integrated with the timely dissemination of these data to those who need to know. The final link in the surveillance chain is the application of these data to prevention and control.'[9]

What does surveillance do?

The key role of surveillance is to identify baseline rates of infection. Deviations from the baseline enable the early recognition of changing patterns of infection and identification of clusters of infection.

> What does surveillance do?
>
> - It identifies baseline rates of infection
> - It identifies deviations from this baseline.

It may also enable identification of changes in risk factors for the infection and can be used to assess the impact of interventions taken to address a particular problem, test new approaches and identify areas for further investigation or research. However, surveillance has further important uses: the provision of quantitative data can be crucial in convincing key hospital staff and decision-makers of the need for action and should be presented regularly to relevant hospital committees as an indicator of the quality of care. The provision of surveillance data places discussions on a factual basis and thus assists in consideration of the need for action and in justifying the need for further resources. It should form part of clinical audit and be embedded in the hospital's clinical governance process. Surveillance data can be important in defence against litigation and to demonstrate that the service is satisfying national standards, for instance, participation in mandatory surveillance and the meeting of targets. The

findings from an active surveillance programme in a hospital should be used routinely in staff education and training to reinforce good practice.

> What are the uses of surveillance?
>
> - Identification of changing patterns of infection and clusters
> - Identification of risk factors for infection
> - Assessment of the impact of interventions to control infection
> - Highlighting of areas warranting further investigation or research
> - Indicator of the quality of care
>   - Demonstration that national standards are being met
>   - Defence in litigation
> - Influencing decision-makers on need for action or resources
> - Education and training.

Sources of data

A strength of MRSA surveillance is that the data are derived from culture of the organism, rather than clinical diagnosis. Not only does this mean firmer diagnosis (microbiological confirmation), but it means that the data are normally concentrated in one area of the hospital, the microbiology laboratory, potentially enabling easier data capture. The data used may result from clinical investigations or active screening of patients and staff and are normally collected as part of alert organism surveillance. As much MRSA carriage is asymptomatic, screening provides important information for control. This may be undertaken at or during admission or on discharge as part of an active programme to control MRSA in particular areas of the hospital where the sequelae of MRSA infection are more serious.[10] Staff screening is usually low yield in terms of identifying MRSA colonisation, as positive samples usually reflect transient colonisation. However, there are certain circumstances where it may be useful and in these circumstances the yield is normally improved by focusing on staff with skin lesions, such as paronychiae or dermatitis. Similarly, there is not a role for routine environmental screening – MRSA is usually found in the environment of positive patients – but it can occasionally be useful in identifying the need to improve cleaning or decontamination procedures.

Objectives, definitions and dataset

The objective of the surveillance needs to be clearly defined in terms of improving the quality of patient care, for instance, reduction in rates of MRSA on a particular ward. It needs to be clear to the staff collecting the data that this serves a useful purpose. Surveillance should be efficient and practical and resources targeted at where an impact can be made. Efficiency and practicality are improved if surveillance needs can be integrated into existing data collection processes, for instance collection of activity data which many hospital units need to undertake routinely. This also encourages participation and completeness of data collection.

The key principles of surveillance include:

- A clear objective related to improving quality of care
- Target it at where an impact can be made
- An agreed case definition, applied systematically and uniformly
- A minimum dataset
- Identification of appropriate data sources
- Practicability – integration as far as possible in to existing data collection processes
- Sufficient accuracy for the purpose
- Consistent collection and reporting of data
- Appropriate analyses and interpretation
- Identification of possible biases in the data
- Timely feedback of information.

A minimum dataset and the process for collecting the data need to be defined. The dataset should include patient and unit identifiers; date of admission for hospital

patients; the date when MRSA was first detected; whether this reflects colonisation or infection; others sites of infection or colonisation; if bacteraemia, the likely source; where MRSA was acquired (hospital, community, specialty, etc.). If MRSA was present on admission, an assessment of whether this was related to previous healthcare contact needs to be undertaken. Differentiating hospital-acquired infection from that acquired outside can be difficult as MRSA infection does not have a delineated incubation period. Infection detected within 2 days of admission is commonly accepted as indicating that infection was acquired prior to the current admission. In these circumstances, it is important to identify whether this reflects acquisition in the same or another hospital or healthcare facility or is true community acquisition. This becomes important when MRSA data are used to compare hospitals and their trajectory towards meeting their target, as infections acquired outside the hospital should be differentiated from hospital acquisitions in the assessment. Ideally, information should be included on the transferring facility, if the MRSA was acquired in another hospital or care home. The antimicrobial susceptibility of the strain is also worthwhile collecting as this may indicate therapeutic options and signal the epidemiological type of the strain, allowing inferences about whether this is the usual strain for that institution or a different one. Other desirable items include the primary diagnosis, an assessment of severity of underlying illnesses, prior antimicrobial therapy, and possible risk factors for infection.

The dataset should include:

- Patient, laboratory, unit/ward and hospital identifiers
- Patient demographics (age, sex)
- Date of admission
- Date of onset of infection (if appropriate)
- Site of the primary infection (if appropriate)

continued on page 135

- Date specimen taken
- Site of specimen (blood culture, wound, *etc.*)
- Where the MRSA was acquired
- Whether part of an outbreak
- Antimicrobial susceptibilities.

Other desirable items include: other sites of MRSA colonisation or infection, date MRSA first detected if colonisation detected before infection, the primary diagnosis, an assessment of severity of underlying illnesses, prior antimicrobial therapy, and possible risk factors for infection.

Quality of the data

The accuracy needs to be sufficient for the purpose of the surveillance. If the data are going to be used for more than simple cluster identification in a particular unit, the quality assumes greater importance. Once hospitals are being compared in national surveillance or the data are the basis for assessment against national targets, it becomes paramount that data collection and reporting are rigorous and consistent with respect to agreed case definitions and underpinning validation of the methods. This means that those responsible for collecting the data should be designated staff, trained in the requirements of consistent data collection.

Numerators, denominators and analysis of the data

The purpose of the surveillance also drives analysis: this should be appropriate to the needs of the target audience. National data requirements may drive local surveillance developments, as in the case of the national targets, now commonplace in the UK. However, even in these circumstances, analyses should be undertaken to meet the needs of the hospital, be it Board or Infection Control Committee members, ward staff and managers, or those involved in the training and induction of clinical and non-clinical staff. The needs of the local hospital usually mean that it is not sufficient to

have hospital-level data, but that it needs to be broken down further to examine the situation in individual units, to assess whether the infections are localised to particular units or more widespread. This will then inform the necessary actions to deal with any problems.

When surveillance is merely being used to track trends in a restricted area such as a ward, it is often sufficient to collect numbers of infections, if the activity on the ward has largely remained unchanged over time. However, the high profile of MRSA means that the data are often used for benchmarking and national targets; in these circumstances, it becomes important to have rates of infection, rather than simply numbers. This then brings in complex issues around appropriate denominators for the infections being counted. Common denominators that are used include the total numbers of specimens tested or admissions or discharges from the relevant area. However, ideally, the denominator should reflect the population at risk as closely as possible, such as the number of in-patient days or device-use days for patients on a critical care unit. This information can be more difficult to collect. In terms of national data, bed occupancy and other hospital episode statistics are often used, which may be constrained by the vagaries of local data entry. Some of these datasets are highly complex and allow the data to be analysed in different ways, for instance with age stratifications or by individual units in a hospital, including intensive care and renal dialysis units. However, this becomes worthless if the local hospital did not input this information accurately.

Recording and monitoring infections

In the same way that the purpose of the surveillance drives its quality and analyses undertaken, it also influences methods for recording and monitoring infections. Simple data recording on file cards or line listings will often serve local purposes and there are infection control packages which can assist with the collation and analysis of surveillance information.[11] Increasingly, statistical methods are used with real-time graphical monitoring showing when numbers of infections are exceeding the normal limits. These are also useful for identifying the effects of interventions on the infection rate. Methods that are increasingly popular are based on those initially developed for industry in the early 20th century to feed back product defect rates to workers as part of maintaining or improving product quality, using statistical process control (SPC) charts. These methods are applicable to many other settings and have been increasingly taken up within healthcare, latterly in epidemiology and infection control, being used to monitor particular HCAI, surgical infection rates, adverse incidents, etc.[12-15] This methodology is very much bound up with continuous quality improvement and is dependent on establishing measures of quality and understanding factors that can affect that quality. The basic principle of the SPC method is that all processes (whether manufacture of products on an assembly line or the factors leading to acquisition of a hospital infection) have inherent variation which can be described statistically. Charts can be set with the appropriate control limits for normal variation based on the unit's past experience, so that deviations from this are apparent and prompt further investigation to explain the cause of this unnatural variation. The charts can also be adjusted to handle a changing situation, for instance, the requirement to drive current levels of MRSA infection downwards. The control limits would then need to be changed to reflect the new target level and practices will need to be changed to move the previously accepted normal endemic rate of infection downwards.

There are a variety of different control charts, of varying levels of sophistication, suitable for different situations. Selection needs to take into account the ease of construction of the chart and interpretation by relevant staff, the statistical distribution of the data, whether dealing with discrete numbers or proportions and the frequency of occurrence of the event

being monitored. Charts like cumulative sum (Cusum) charts or exponentially weighted moving average charts may be more sensitive to small changes, but often have the drawback that they are more difficult to construct and interpret. The Shewhart *c*-chart is that commonly used in hospitals to monitor and feed back infection rates, a major advantage being the ease of interpretation and virtual real-time feedback (Fig. 16.3). This can be valuable in giving more ownership and responsibility for infection control to ward staff. Moving average charts can be useful for monitoring the national picture and movement towards the target level.

Feeding back the data and action

Most importantly, the data need to be fed back to those involved in the data collection in a way that is relevant to them, so as to maintain their interest in participating in the surveillance. For the data to be of local use, feedback must be timely. It is important that potential biases in the data are identified and included in the feedback, for instance changes in reporting or diagnostic methods during a particular period. Whether such assessment biases matter depends on what the data are used for. The bias matters less when the data are being used to detect a change (if the number reporting properly are relatively constant), but becomes important when the data are being used for benchmarking purposes or to assess practice.

Although the SENIC study[8] showed that merely feeding back the data resulted in improvements in infection rates, the data need to be part of quality improvement and the clinical governance process of the hospital, integral to its prioritisation procedures. This means that there should be designated senior staff in individual hospital directorates with responsibility to act on the results. In some hospitals, these responsibilities are now being built into staff job plans and performance appraisal. Methods being used to examine the data to bring about change include treating

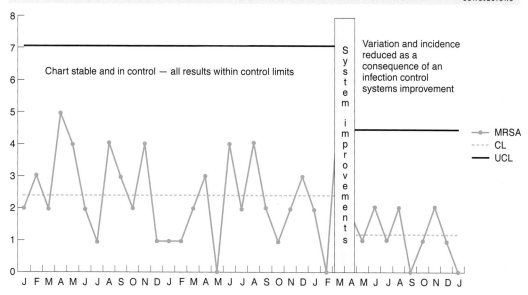

Figure 16.3
Statistical process control chart showing new MRSA acquisitions on a ward by month, before and after the introduction of system improvements (source E. Curran). CL, control limit; UCL, upper control limit.

each new case as an untoward incident, with investigation of possible root causes for the infection (Fig. 16.4).

Resourcing the surveillance

Robust surveillance of MRSA, or indeed of HCAI generally, is not free of expense. Significant resources are required in terms of staffing to co-ordinate surveillance, train designated staff in consistent data collection, undertake analyses and interpretation of the data, and prepare information for dissemination to key staff. These costs may be considerable, but the evidence indicates that the benefits outweigh the costs. The cost–benefit analysis of the SENIC study showed that only about 6% of hospital acquired infections would need to be prevented to offset the cost of the infection control programme, which included surveillance (the expectation was that 30% of the infections were preventable). More recently the Department of Health's 'Going further faster' guidance included a tool for estimating the costs of MRSA bacteraemia and

potential savings from meeting national target reductions in trusts plus examples from English trusts of significant savings already made.[16] Some trusts have benefited by receiving discounts on their contributions to the Clinical Negligence Scheme for Trusts as a result of demonstrating their active surveillance activities.

Conclusions

MRSA surveillance is key to the control of MRSA, as demonstrated by national programmes to drive down MRSA rates based on targets set through the surveillance data. Surveillance is not only central to the infection control programme, but is an indicator of the quality of care and also fundamental to the hospital's clinical governance. It will only be effective if based on sound principles and robust timely data. Surveillance linked to quality improvement needs to be driven at hospital level by influential staff with the support of senior management. Robust surveillance needs resourcing, but the benefits outweigh the costs.

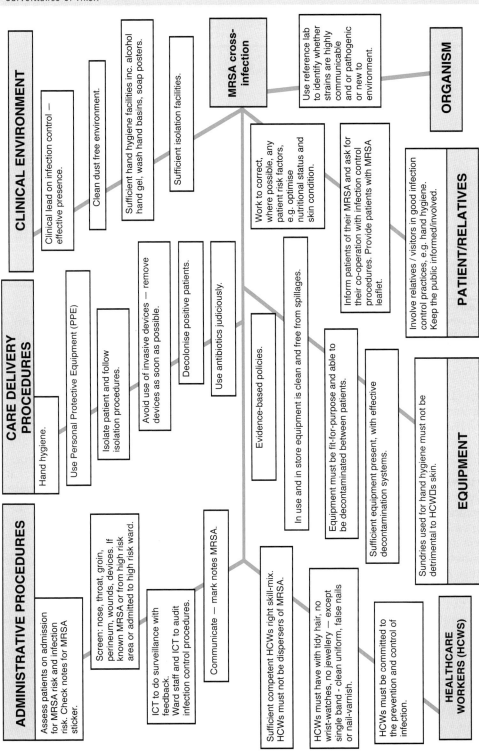

Figure 16.4
Fishbone cause and effect diagram showing the factors that impact on transmission of MRSA (source E. Curran).

References

1. European Antimicrobial Resistance Surveillance System [Online]. Annual Report 2004 [cited 27 June 2006]. Available at: <http://www.rivm.nl/earss/result/Monitoring_reports/Annual_reports.jsp>.

2. Department of Health. *Winning Ways: working together to reduce healthcare associated infection in England*. London: Department of Health, December 2003.

3. Report by the Comptroller and Auditor General. Improving patient care by reducing the risk of hospital acquired infection: a progress report. London: The Stationery Office. HC 876 session 2003–2004: 14 July 2004.

4. Department of Health. Bloodborne MRSA infection rates to be halved by 2008 - Reid (*press release*). London: Department of Health, Thursday 4 November 2004 [cited 27 June 2006]. Available at: <http://www.dh.gov.uk/PublicationsAndStatistics/PressReleases/PressReleasesNotices/fs/en?CONTENT_ID=4093533&chk=MY%2BkD/>.

5. MRSA surveillance system – results. Available on Department of Health's website [cited 27 June 2006] at: <http://www.dh.gov.uk/PublicationsAndStatistics/Publications/PublicationsStatistics/PublicationsStatisticsArticle/fs/en?CONTENT_ID=4085951&chk=HBt2QD>.

6. Healthcare associated infections – a strategy for hospitals in Wales. Public Health Protection Division. Welsh Assembly Government. July 2004 [cited 27 June 2006]. Available at: <http://www.cmo.wales.gov.uk/content/publications/strategies/healthcare-associated-infections-e.pdf>.

7. Scottish surveillance of healthcare associated infection programme. Quarterly report on meticillin resistant *Staphylococcus aureus* bacteraemias in Scotland. January 2001 – December 2005 [cited 27 June 2006]. Available at: <http://www.show.scot.nhs.uk/scieh/infectious/hai/MRSA_quarter_reports/MRSAApr06/MRSAApr06.pdf>.

8. Haley RW, Culver DH, White JW *et al*. The efficacy of infection surveillance and control programs in preventing nosocomial infections in US hospitals. *Am J Epidemiol* 1984; **121**: 182.

9. Thacker SB, Berkelman RL. Public health surveillance in the United States. *Epidemiol Rev* 1988; **10**: 164–90.

10. Coia JE, Duckworth GJ, Edwards DI *et al*.: for the Joint Working Party of the British Society of Antimicrobial Chemotherapy, the Hospital Infection Society, and the Infection Control Nurses Association. Guidelines for the control and prevention of meticillin-resistant *Staphylococcus aureus* (MRSA) in healthcare facilities. *J Hosp Infect* 2006; **63 (Suppl 1)**: 1–44.

11. Health Protection Agency. Infection control IT implementation and evaluation project. Report prepared for the Department of Health, August 2005 [cited 27 June 2006]. Available at: <http://www.hpa.org.uk/infections/topics_az/hai/ICITIAE_report_Dec_2005.pdf>.

12. Sellick Jr JA. The use of statistical process control charts in hospital epidemiology. *Infect Control Hosp Epidemiol* 1993; **14**: 649–56.

13. Benneyan JC. Statistical quality control methods in infection control and hospital epidemiology, part I: introduction and basic theory. *Infect Control Hosp Epidemiol* 1998; **19**: 194–214.

14. Benneyan JC. Statistical quality control methods in infection control and hospital epidemiology, part II: chart use, statistical properties, and research issues. *Infect Control Hosp Epidemiol* 1998; **19**: 256–83.

15. Curran ET, Benneyan JC, Hood J. Controlling methicillin-resistant *Staphylococcus aureus*: a feedback approach using annotated statistical process control charts. *Infect Control Hosp Epidemiol* 2002; **23**: 13–8.

16. Department of Health. Going further faster: implementing the Saving Lives delivery programme. London: Department of Health, 9 May 2006 [cited 27 June 2006]. Available at: <http://www.dh.gov.uk/PublicationsAndStatistics/Publications/PublicationsPolicyAndGuidance/PublicationsPolicyAndGuidanceArticle/fs/en?CONTENT_ID=4134547&chk=oIl1eR>.

Index

Page numbers in *italics* refer to information that is shown only in a table or diagram.

abscesses 68, 69, 75
accessory genes 24–5
AccuProbe SA Culture Identification Test 52
airborne transmission 103
ambulances 114–15
aminoglycosides 63–4
animals, MRSA in 42–4
antibiotics
  for MRSA *80*
  newer 65
  properties *83*
  resistance 59–65
  susceptibility testing 53
artesunate 93
arthritis, septic 75

BacLite Rapid MRSA 56
bacteraemia 69, 73–4, 131
bacterial interference 97–8
bacteriophage therapy 96–7
Barber's Law 6
BBL Crystal MRSA ID System 54
berberine 94
biochemical identification kits 52
blood cultures confirmation 55
bone infection 69, 75
borderline resistance 51
BURST 23

carriers
  isolation 120–1
  search for 118
  silent pool 119–20
  treatment and follow-up 115–16
cathelicidin 15
cefoxitin 53
celbenin 3
chemotaxis inhibiting protein 16

chlorhexidene 88–9, 115
chromogenic media 53–4
cleaning 101–7
  effect 106
clindamycin 63
clinical risk assessment 119, 122
clinics 114
clones 25, 26, 110
  new 110–11
cloxacillin 6
colonisation 71–3
  consequences 87–8
  eradication 89
  increase 118–21
  management 90–*91*
  mucosal 16–17
  patient factors *87*
  postoperative risk factors *76*
community
  control 109–16
  risk factors *109*
community-acquired MRSA 27, 30–1, 37–47
  clinical features 67–70
  infection diagnosis 70
  likely patients *72*
community-onset MRSA 39
confirmation
  1 day 52–3
  rapid 54–5
contamination in hospitals 104
cross-infection reduction 121
CytAMP MRSA assay 55

dataset 134
day-care centres 114
decolonisation 87–91
  agents 88–9
  infection strategies 89–90

decontamination 84–5
definitions in SISS guidance *123*
detection 111–12
  in diagnostic laboratories 6
drug abusers, parenteral 40

EARSS 8
EARSS project 30
EMRSA 8, 10, 26–7
  current clones 26–7
endocarditis 74–5
enrichment culture 52
epidemigenicity 8
epidemiology 29–35, 39–41
  in community 109–11
  staphylococcal 102
essential oils 94
Etest method 53
EVIGENE MRSA Detection Kit 54–5
evolution 21–8
  history 25–7
extracellular adherence protein 15

Fishbone cause and effect diagram 138
flucloxacillin 61, 79, 80
fluoroquinolones 64
food animals 43–4
furunculosis 68

garlic 96
genome, core 24–5
GenoType MRSA Direct 56
geographic variation 30
glycopeptides 61–2, 80–1
glycylcyclines 83

hand hygiene 111
hand-touch sites 106
home care 113–14
honey 96
hospital-acquired MRSA 39, 71
  vs community-acquired MRSA *110*
hospitals
  cleaning 101–7
  MRSA spread factors *29*
household pets 43
hyperforin 94
Hyplex StaphyloResist 56

IDI MRSA 56–7
immune system
  cellular immunity 16
  humoral immunity 16
  innate evasion 15–16
immunocapture-coupled PCR 56
immunotherapy, passive 17
in silico analysis 24
infections
  antibiotics for *80*
  clinical presentation 71–8
  control practice 121–2
  disseminated 69
  MRSA associated 73–6
  postoperative 75–6
  recording and monitoring 135–6
  rise in The Netherlands 31
  rise in Scandinavia 31
  rise in UK 31
  treatment 79–86
inflammatory local responses 16–17
interference therapy 17

joint infections 69
  prosthetic 75

kindergartens 114

laboratory detection and confirmation 51–8
laboratory reporting 49–50, 51–3
  next day 53–5
  same-day 55–7
β-lactamases 60–1, 79
latex agglutination tests 52
linezolid 1–2
lipopeptides 82–3

macrolides 63
mecA 21, 23–4, 38, 50–1
  detection 55
medicinal plants 94
methicillin
  history 4
  MICs 5
  molecular basis of resistance 50–1
  replacements 21
methicillin-resistant *Staphylococcus aureus* see
  MRSA

methicillin-susceptible *Staphylococcus aureus see*
    MSSA
minimum inhibitory concentrations 5, 6
MLS resistance 63
molecular basis, methicillin resistance 50–1
MRSA 38–44
    carriage 31–2
    cf MSSA 17–18
    epidemic *see* EMRSA
    Group III 7
    historical perspective 3–12
    outbreaks 3
    rate factors *29*
    rate variation 29–30
MRSA-Screen PBP2a latex agglutination 54
MSSA 13
    cf MRSA 17–18
multilocus sequence typing 22–3
mupirocin 9, 65, 88–9, 115

nafcillin 79
necrotising fasciitis 68
neonatal toxic shock 15
nursing homes 112–13
nursing management 123–5

osteomyelitis 69, 75
oxacillin 3
oxazolidinones 10, 81–2
Panton-Valentine leukocidin 15, 25, 38, 110
patients, admission management 122–5,
    126–7
PCR assay 55, 56
penicillin binding protein 7, 21, 50, 60–1, 79
peptides 14–15
peptidoglycan 14
phytomedicines 94
pigs 44
pneumonia 68–9
    hospital/ventilator acquired 75
polysaccharides 14
prevalence 37
prevention
    CA-MRSA 41–2
    CO-MRSA 42
Public Health Laboratory Service 3
public transport 114–15
pulmonary infections 68–9

pulsed field gel electrophoresis 22, 60
purpura fulminans 69
pyomyositis 68
pyrogenic toxin superantigens 15

recombination, low frequency 25
rifampicin 64
risk factors 72

sandalwood oil 94
scalded skin syndrome 25
SCC*mec* 23–4, 26, 38–9, 61
schools 114
Scottish Infection Standards and Strategy Group
    117–25
Screening
    for carriage 84
    targeted 119
SENIC study 132, 136
SENTRY programme *30*
septic shock 69
Shewhart *c*-chart 136
skin and soft tissue infections 68, 73
sodium fusidate 64
SSA*mec* 110
staff screening 125
Staphychrom II 52
Staphylococcus aureus
    carriage 103
    infection frequency 73
    infectious syndromes 13–19
    survival 104
    transmission cycle 102
    virulence factors 14–15
streptogramins 82
surveillance 32–3, 131–9
    data sources 133–4
    principles 134
    role 133
swabs 112

tampon-associated disease 15
taxis 114–15
tea-tree oil 95
tefibazumab 17
teicoplanin 10, 11, 62, 80–1
tetracyclines 64
toxic-shock syndrome 25

transmission
  human 104–5
  staphylococcal, dynamic 105
treatment
  alternative 93–100
  considerations 83–4
trimethoprim 65
tube coagulase test 52

USA, MRSA situation 30–1

vaccines 17

vanA complex 62
vancomycin 4, 9–10, 11, 61–2, 80–1
  reduced susceptibility 27
Velogene Rapid MRSA assay 54
ventilator-associated pneumonia 75
virulence gene expression 14
VISA 31, 62
VRSA 31

wall teichoic acids 14–15
Wenzel, Richard 6–7

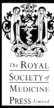
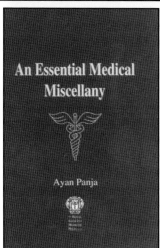

Putting you first

starts with joining us

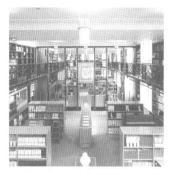

Attend specialty meetings, seminars and conferences around the UK...

read and research...

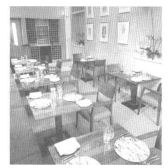

entertain at the bar or enjoy a meal at the restaurant ...

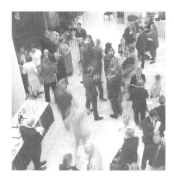

gain accreditation...

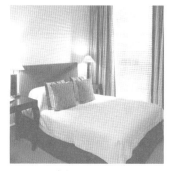

stay overnight...

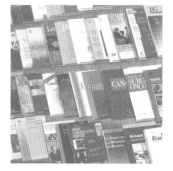

Receive medical title discounts and paper or online JRSM...

The Royal Society of Medicine's commitment to the 'exchange of information and ideas on the science, practice and organisation of medicine' is over 200 years old.

Today, this heritage is sharply focused on the needs of medical practitioners in a pressurised and demanding world.

That is why the RSM offers you the satisfaction of broadening medical horizons across diverse specialisations as well as the pleasure of good company, comfortable surroundings and club facilities.

We would be delighted if you could join us.

Membership starts from £30 a year.

For more information contact the membership team on +44 (0)20 7290 2991 or membership@rsm.ac.uk or visit www.rsmmembership.org

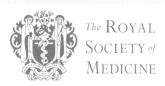

The ROYAL SOCIETY of MEDICINE

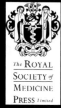
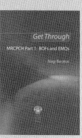
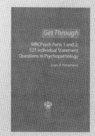